The
EVERYTHING®
Body Shaping Book

Dear Reader:

You may have picked up this book because of the promise made on the front cover: You can change the shape of your body! We have taken the best of the various programs out there and combined them into one easy-to-follow plan with that one goal in mind. If you read this book and follow the suggestions and program in it, you *can* actually change the shape of your body by concentrating on the trouble parts, one at a time, and applying the principles of body shaping as outlined in this book.

As you do this program you will find that there are a number of other benefits you will enjoy just by following this body-shaping method. For example, in addition to watching your appearance improve, you will quickly notice that your mood is better, you are sleeping better, your energy levels are increasing, you are tolerating stress better, and you just look and feel better overall. Now, who wouldn't want to give that promise a chance? Try it and see. What have you got to lose (except some weight, fatigue, and scrawny arms)?

Good luck,

Katie McBride   *Lesley Bolton*

The EVERYTHING® Series

Editorial

Publishing Director	Gary M. Krebs
Managing Editor	Kate McBride
Copy Chief	Laura MacLaughlin
Acquisitions Editor	Bethany Brown
Production Editor	Khrysti Nazzaro
	Jamie Wielgus
Technical Reviewer	Jonny Bowden, M.A., C.N., C.N.S.

Production

Production Director	Susan Beale
Production Manager	Michelle Roy Kelly
Series Designers	Daria Perreault
	Colleen Cunningham
Cover Design	Paul Beatrice
	Frank Rivera
Layout and Graphics	Colleen Cunningham
	Rachael Eiben
	Michelle Roy Kelly
	Daria Perreault
	Erin Ring
Cover Art	Marcy Ramsey
Photographer	Deborah Boardman
Models	Mary Varaitis
	Erica Cava

Visit the entire Everything® Series at everything.com

THE
EVERYTHING
BODY SHAPING BOOK

Sculpt your body to perfection—tone your
thighs, abs, hips, arms, legs, and more!

Kate McBride & Lesley Bolton

A

Adams Media
Avon, Massachusetts

This book is dedicated to strong women everywhere, particularly my daughter Caitlin, who has been a constant source of inspiration and strength.

An Everything® Series Book.
Everything® and everything.com® are registered trademarks of F+W Publications, Inc.

Published by Adams Media,
an F+W Publications Company
57 Littlefield Street, Avon, MA 02322 U.S.A.
www.adamsmedia.com

ISBN: 1-58062-977-6
Printed in the United States of America.

J I H G F E D C B A

Library of Congress Cataloging-in-Publication Data
available from publisher

*This book is available at quantity discounts for bulk purchases.
For information, call 1-800-872-5627.*

Contents

Acknowledgments

A huge and heartfelt thank you—

to Bethany for her infinite patience and her uncompromising commitment to quality.

to Laura for her all-around goodwill and her endless supply of editorial bandages.

and to Lesley for stellar performance above and beyond the call of duty.

Thanks for all your help! Remember, "what doesn't kill you makes you stronger."

I want to also acknowledge the early "pioneers"—those who showed us that a woman who worked out with weights could be strong, and still feminine and beautiful: Rachel McLish, Gladys Portugues, Cory Everson, and Joyce Vedral.

Kate

Top Ten Benefits
of Body Shaping

1. Tone, strengthen, and sculpt the muscles of problem areas for definition and beauty.
2. Increased energy levels.
3. Prevent or delay osteoporosis by increasing bone density.
4. Increased self-esteem and self-confidence.
5. Relieve stress.
6. Increased endurance and muscle strength.
7. Increased metabolic rate.
8. Improved posture.
9. Live a longer and more satisfying life.
10. Offset the negative effects of menopause.

Introduction

▶WHAT PERSON DOESN'T WANT to change at least one part of his or her body? Even those fortunate enough to have a great shape, whether they obtained it from nature or by hard work, probably still have misgivings about one body part or another. One person may complain about her hips, another about her abs, and another about her small calves. Diet and exercise are generally accepted as the most effective methods for changing your body for a very good reason—because they both work, and work best in combination. A dedicated program of regular exercise and a healthy diet will go a long way in helping you to obtain the body of your dreams. However, no matter how hard you work and how well you stick to your food program, there are certain changes to your body that cannot be obtained through diet and exercise alone.

For example, perhaps you have small calves and you think that your legs do not look well proportioned because they are larger and thicker at your thighs and straight and thin at your lower legs. Obviously, diet can do nothing about this body problem, and exercise, while going a long way toward contributing to overall muscularity and shapeliness, actually will not do anything to reshape your calves. However, if you follow the simple calf program outlined in this book, you can reshape your calves to make them toned, muscular, and shapely within a matter of a few months.

Or, maybe you are plagued with a chest that is smaller than you would like. Short of implants or padded bras, you may think there is nothing you can do about this feature, or should we say *lack* of one. Well, you would be partially correct. While nothing you will read in this book will actually make your breasts larger, there are things you can do that will build up the muscles under the breasts and build a line down the center of the breasts that will create both a look of lift and the illusion of cleavage. Perhaps your upper arms are your problem. It is that annoying little excess skin on the back of the upper arm that "waves" every time you lift your arm. Again, diet won't touch this problem and your general exercise program will not solve it either. But targeted exercise will. Targeted exercise is what this book is about. The body-shaping program presented here will allow you to target your problem areas and work on fixing them.

The program presented in this book is called "body shaping" because by following it, you can actually reshape different parts of your body, one at a time, to create the total body look you desire. Imagine yourself as an artist with a paintbrush who creates a work of art by painting one area at a time until all the parts come together to produce the finished look. It is the same with the body-shaping program: While you achieve overall fitness by exercising, you are also concentrating on one body part at a time, focusing on that body part and making it look the way you want it to by using particular exercise movements.

The program is simple—each chapter takes one area of your body and presents a set of exercises based on the principles of resistance training. Most of the exercises in this book use light weights for resistance because this is the most effective way to create shape and form. You can choose just the body parts you want to fix or you can create a total body program by doing two exercises for each body part from each chapter. Either way, you are on the way to doing something about those annoying parts of your body that have always caused you frustration.

Try this program for six weeks and see if you don't agree that it offers an easy and effective answer to whatever has been bothering you about your shape. Remember, diet and exercise are important for obtaining your overall fitness goals but only body shaping can change the shape of your body! Ⓔ

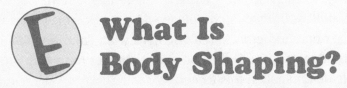

Chapter 1

What Is Body Shaping?

Body shaping is for anyone who wants to reshape certain problem areas of her or his body. It is not a weight-loss program, nor is it a program meant to create massive bulky muscle. It simply targets specific problem areas of the body and gives you solutions for those problems!

The Battle of the Bulge

Everyone battles the bulge, even those men and women plastered all over television, movies, and advertisements. Don't think for one moment that anyone has a quick-fix solution for toning and sculpting the body. If such a thing existed, everyone would have the "ideal" body—which of course doesn't even exist. Each person's body is different; therefore, *the* ideal can only be *your* ideal. Battling the bulge with body shaping does take work. It doesn't have to be backbreaking hard work (and, yes, it can even be fun!), but it does require you to be active and set forth with an unquenchable determination to succeed.

Understanding Fat

When going into battle, you stand a much better chance of success if you know your enemy. If battling the bulge is your reason for picking up this book, then you must get to know your fat. First of all, you can never be fat-free, so give up that dream now. Your body needs fat.

If you are a woman, your body needs more fat than a man's body needs. On average, a woman will have twice the amount of fat that a man has. Women are at yet another disadvantage. Women tend to store fat in the lower region of the body (hips, butt, and thighs), whereas men tend to store fat in the upper region of the body. You guessed it: It's harder to lose body fat from the lower region of the body. But don't despair; it can be done.

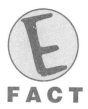

FACT

The body mass index (BMI) is a common tool used to determine a person's body fat based on his or her height and weight. You can calculate your BMI at ✎*www.caloriecontrol.org/bmi.html*. However, keep in mind that this is only an estimate. If you are muscular, this calculation will be slightly off as muscle weighs more than fat.

Your body must maintain a certain percentage of body fat to function properly. Fat is very beneficial in several ways. For instance, fat cushions your organs. Without it, your organs could easily be damaged. Fat gives your hair shine and keeps your skin smooth. Fat also aids a woman's reproductive system and provides the energy needed to nourish a fetus. Fat isn't all bad. Don't attack fat, battle the bulge—the excess fat.

Don't Go for the Gimmicks

In your attempt to win the weight war, you may have been tempted by one or several of the thousands of weight-loss body-shaping products out on the market. Don't buy it! The only thing you'll lose is your money. While it is certainly wonderful to dream of losing 30 pounds in just two weeks or getting six-pack abs in just three days, it is just a dream. Everyone would love a quick fix and companies and individuals prey on that desire. The billion-dollar industry proves it. There's a reason there are so many pills, programs, and solutions for quick and easy weight loss and muscle tone readily available on the market: Not one has proved its ability to make you lose weight, tone muscle, be healthy, and maintain your ideal shape. This isn't to say that you *won't* be able to lose weight, tone muscle, be healthy, and maintain your ideal shape. It's just going to take more work than popping a pill.

The battle of the bulge can only be won with time, patience, determination, dedication, and work. Physicians, nutritionists, and fitness experts worldwide have been saying for years that the best way to get your body into shape is to eat well and exercise. Something so simple is often quickly given up on in favor of the "wonder drugs." Don't fall prey to the gimmicks. Be smart and give the only tried-and-true method a shot.

Body shaping will help you win the battle of the bulge, while maintaining both physical and mental health. It will help you achieve that ideal body shape you've only dreamed of. It will give you what those weight-loss body-shaping products promised but could not deliver: a happy, healthy, in-shape you.

The Difference Between Weight Loss and Body Shaping

When people think of shaping their bodies, many immediately think of losing weight. While some weight loss does occur, weight loss and body shaping are not synonymous. Weight loss is when you get on the bathroom scale and jump for joy at having lost a few pounds. Body shaping is an exercise regimen designed to help you sculpt and tone your muscles, which leads to a fit and trim figure.

Obsession with Weight

More and more people are becoming obsessed with their weight. No one's body is perfect, but everyone thinks it should be. And most believe the way to achieve the perfect body is to lose weight. Just take a look at the men and women who've made it to the spotlight. Several runway models and movie stars look as though they don't have an ounce of fat on them. But take a closer look; some don't seem to have much muscle either.

When a person becomes obsessed with losing weight, often the obsession leads to doing whatever it takes to shed the pounds—excessively exercising, going on crash diets, starving the body, and the list goes on and on. When a person becomes so focused on the weight aspect of their physical appearance, he or she loses sight of the fitness and strength aspects of the body. All that matters to them is that one number on the scale.

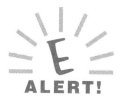

ALERT!

Never, ever assume that starving yourself will help you achieve your ideal body shape. The only way to lose weight and get fit is to exercise and eat well. Notice that "eat" is part of the formula.

Hide the Scales

You are going to learn to shape and sculpt your body, creating a healthy and strong physical appearance. Your very first task is to hide the scales. Stick them in the basement, an out-of-reach cabinet, under your son's bed, or in any other place you aren't likely to want to visit. Next, try to forget where you hid them. Better yet, have a family member or friend hide the scales for you. You are not allowed to constantly jump on the scale and let your weight affect your mood and/or motivation during body shaping.

Try to put the thought of weight out of your mind. It doesn't matter here. What does matter is strengthening the muscles, becoming physically fit, and reducing the amount of body fat while increasing the amount of muscle. After following this program for a few weeks you may be convinced that you are losing weight because you can fit into clothes you couldn't before, your legs feel tighter and toned, and you can actually see a slimmer but more shapely body in the mirror. However, if you get on the scale you may find that your weight has actually not changed! How can that be? It is because muscle weighs more than fat, so while you are reshaping your body and it looks better, you are not actually losing weight.

Don't Just Diet—Body Shape!

If you simply can't help thinking about weight loss, that's okay. You certainly aren't alone. However, it is still a good idea to hide the scales, at least until you begin to see changes in your physical appearance. Those visual changes will help offset any disappointment or frustration you may be feeling with your weight-loss efforts.

You Need the Exercise

Many people turn to dieting as the primary means of losing weight despite the well-known fact that any successful weight-loss effort must be supplemented by a regular program of exercise and physical activity. A recent study documented that an hour of exercise daily is required for successful weight loss. It is not enough just to cut calories; one must participate in a dedicated program of physical activity in order to create permanent and positive changes to the body. A combination of dieting and exercise is the answer for those who want to achieve real changes in the overall appearance of their body.

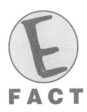

The fact is, once you begin body shaping, you are likely to gain a little weight. This isn't a bad thing! Muscle weighs more than fat, and since you will be building muscle, it is likely you will see some weight gain.

Combine a Good Diet with Body Shaping

There is a big difference between dieting and body shaping. Dieting, a carefully designed reduction in the amount of calories, fat, or carbohydrates consumed, will help you lose weight but is not the answer to every figure problem. This book is *not* about dieting—more than enough has been written about various diets. This book focuses on body shaping, the act of getting your body into physical shape by toning and sculpting the muscles to help you conquer every figure problem. You can accomplish weight loss if you pick a diet that works for you, follow it with dedication, and combine it with the body-shaping program offered here.

Sculpting the Body, Part by Part

In this book, we are targeting specific problem areas, one at a time. We will provide you with a series of movements and exercises that will actually reshape each body part. For the most part, the type of exercise technique used will be weight-training movements, simply because weight training is the fastest and most effective means of reshaping the body, but we will offer a combination of different exercise techniques to make up the program.

What Is Weight Training?

Weight training is a method of building muscle strength and endurance over time through the use of resistance in progressively increasing amounts. Weight training is not the same as bodybuilding, which is a competitive sport. Weight training is muscle conditioning that can be adapted to every body's needs. When you condition your muscles, you train to increase muscle strength or muscle or both. Weight training uses resistance to achieve this conditioning response. Since weight training conditions the specific muscles that have been challenged, it is the perfect method to apply when you are concentrating on particular body parts.

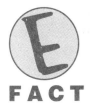

FACT

For a while, running was all the craze, later to be supplanted by aerobics, step aerobics, stair-stepping, jogging, walking, and finally yoga and Pilates. Through it all, a dedicated core group of fitness enthusiasts were committed to the philosophy that working out with weights is the most effective means to body fitness.

A Program with Many Names

Also known as strength training, resistance training, or, at its most serious and intense levels, bodybuilding, working out with weights experienced a surge in popularity during the 1990s, as more and more women became convinced of the dramatic results possible by following a solid and sensible weight-training program. Women's magazines started to include photos of women in workout gear with a variety of gleaming silver dumbbells strewn around on the ground. Gone was the "twiggy" look of the earlier decades and in was the strong, sexy look of women like Linda Hamilton in *The Terminator*, Madonna, and even Angelina Jolie as Lara Croft of *Tomb Raider*.

The reality is that women discovered what men have known for a long time—that training with weights can reshape the body faster and more effectively than any other exercise method. Not only are weights faster and more effective, but they also have one other advantage over other fitness programs—the ability to target specific areas of the body, isolate the muscle group, and concentrate on reshaping or sculpting that specific body part. Since muscle is more dense than fat, it can firm the hips, thighs, and backs of the upper arms, areas that running and aerobics can't help no matter how much you do.

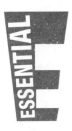

ESSENTIAL

As you are reading, imagine your ideal body shape. It is important to keep your mind focused on your goals as you perform these exercises. The mind is a very important tool used in body shaping. You might as well start exercising it now.

Thus, body shaping was born, as well as a subset of it, spot sculpting. With an applied program of working out with weights, you can succeed in reshaping your entire body or choose to concentrate on specific problem areas and sculpt them to perfection.

Adding Muscle to Create Shape

Weight training is also known as progressive resistance training. Progressive resistance refers to the process of gradually increasing the overload placed on the muscle. Systematic progressive resistance makes the muscle stronger, improves its tone, and increases its mass. Advanced training routines gradually increase the resistance by using a combination of methods, including increasing the amount of weight used, increasing the repetitions performed, or even by decreasing the amount of rest time between sets.

Muscle strength refers to the maximum amount of weight your muscles can lift in one repetition. Training to develop strength uses heavy weights for few repetitions to reach muscle failure. Muscle endurance refers to a muscle's ability to continually lift weight over a period of time. Training to develop endurance is achieved by lifting lighter weights for more repetitions.

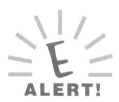

ALERT!

People often don't realize that it's possible to be both thin and fat. A person may be small in size, yet have a very low percentage of lean body mass.

Even if you are someone who already has a regular fitness regimen such as running, aerobics, or regular participation in a sport such as tennis or swimming, you still may not be happy with the pocket of loose skin at the back of your upper arm or your soft abs. Or perhaps you are thin, but do not have the definitive muscle tone you desire. For example, consider an average-sized woman who does not have a weight problem, but is still unhappy with the shape of her body. Perhaps it is just straight like a pole with no curves or shape. Using the program in this book will enable her to increase the size of her muscles and therefore create a shape and curve where there was none before. What is important to remember in body shaping is that it's not the size or shape of the body that matters, it's the relationship of lean mass to fat mass.

Spot Reducing: Myth or Reality?

You may reduce your overall body size by diet but only exercise will tone and firm the body parts. Haven't you ever seen someone who loses an enormous amount of weight through dieting but who still has an unattractive body shape because he or she is soft and flabby? Dieting must be supplemented with an exercise routine in order to achieve real body changes.

This book is based on the premise that working out with weights is the most effective program to choose for the exercise portion of your body-shaping plan. If weight training is used, muscles are formed and they provide shape and curves under the skin at the same time that the fat is melting away. The idea is to build in curves and firm flesh where you want it rather than just settling for being thinner but shapeless. Working out with weights is the perfect way to target the spots you want to build and make that happen!

For example, concentrating on building muscle on the shoulders and the upper back (see the deltoid exercises and latissimus dorsi exercises in Chapters 8 and 11) will change the entire look of your upper body. By broadening the shoulders and the lats, you will create a wider line across the top of your body (the upper end of the classic "hourglass figure") and also create the illusion of a smaller waist. Imagine the letter V, with your shoulders being the top of the letter and your waist being the point at the bottom—the broader your shoulders, the smaller your waist looks!

Spot reducing is also the best method for dealing with those problem areas such as the thighs and buttocks. No amount of dieting will change saddlebag thighs, but working the surrounding muscles of the legs such as the quadriceps and biceps will tighten the entire area and change the shape to a tighter, more toned look—again, proof that body shaping can do what dieting cannot.

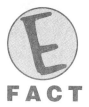

FACT

Working the calf muscles will not only create a shapelier lower leg but will affect the look of the entire leg by adding better proportion and detracting from the larger size of the upper leg. Instead of just having "table legs" (straight up and down from the knee to the ankle) you will now have strong, shapely, muscular legs.

Side Benefits of This Program

In addition to the fast physical changes you'll see, there are other benefits to body shaping. For instance, body shaping increases bone density and therefore plays a dramatic role in preventing or delaying osteoporosis. Gradual bone loss begins in both men and women between the ages of thirty and fifty. When you body shape to build muscle, you are also building bone. The exercise stimulates the bone tissue and causes stress and tension on the bone, triggering small electrical currents that tell the bone to repair and regenerate.

In a recent study, menopausal and postmenopausal women who performed some high-intensity strength-training exercises twice a week for one year had measurable increases in spinal and hip bone density. The group that did not exercise lost 2.5 percent density from the hip and 1.8 percent from the spine, on average.

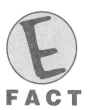

FACT

Regular exercise with weights goes a long way to offset the negative effects of menopause. Exercise not only helps to increase bone mass and reduce the effects of osteoporosis, it can help ease the problems of poor circulation, insomnia, and depression that often bother menopausal women.

Improve Your Posture

Another added benefit is a natural improvement in overall posture. You will note that there are frequent reminders about positioning your body as you go through the exercise routines in this book. It is necessary to assume the correct form in order for these exercises to have their full effectiveness. After a few weeks of practicing these exercises, you will notice that you are unconsciously assuming this correct form even when you are not working out. The reminders to "roll back your shoulders" or "tuck in your stomach" become second nature and after a while you will become aware whenever your back is not straight or your shoulders are tense or not rolled back. Improper posture will actually become almost uncomfortable. You will find yourself standing and sitting straighter with an added awareness of your overall posture.

Improve the Quality of Life

There are several ways in which body shaping can improve the overall quality of your life. For instance, once you establish an exercise routine, you will find that you have increased energy levels. You won't feel as fatigued and will find that you have the energy to do those things you always wanted to do but put off because you're too tired.

As you build up muscle tone and notice the visible difference in your appearance, your self-esteem and self-confidence will rise. You'll find that you not only look great, but feel great, too. You'll be able to accomplish more with ease since you will be stronger than you once were. Who knows? You may even take up new hobbies and participate in more activities.

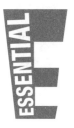

Of course, building your body's strength will also allow you to have more fun by improving your endurance. You will be able to do those activities that bring you the greatest pleasure for longer periods of time.

Body shaping will also help you relieve stress. Everyone faces stress on a daily basis, but it is those that are able to relieve their stress in healthy ways that come out ahead. Physical exercise will help you release pent-up frustrations. In turn, reducing the amount of stress you endure will help you to sleep better at night. You will wake refreshed and ready to face the upcoming day. Ⓔ

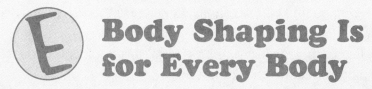

Chapter 2

Body Shaping Is for Every Body

Whether you are overweight or just want to tone and tighten specific parts of your body, this book can give you what you need. You will be able to design a program that uses exercises for every body part for an overall, total body effect or focus on particular sections to target troublesome areas.

Who This Book Is For

First of all, shut the blinds and the door, take off all your clothes, and take a long hard look in the mirror. Don't try to suck in your stomach or stand at an angle that hides those areas you'd rather not see. Remember, the blinds and door are closed; no one else is going to see you. Slowly turn around, trying to see your body from every angle. Now, is there any part of your body that you would like to change? That is, is there any part of your body that you would like to flatten, tone up, broaden, or slim down? Whether there is just one or several, this book is for you. (Okay, you can put your clothes back on now.)

For the Beginner

Beginners and more experienced fitness enthusiasts alike will be able to use the exercises and ideas offered in this book to their advantage. For those of you just beginning your personal body-shaping endeavor, this program is a great way to ease into the world of physical fitness. While you will be offered advice and recommended exercises to use, building the program is up to you. This means that you needn't be worried about starting off with too much too fast. Once you become comfortable with the level you have started with, you always have the option of adding more to the program to take it up a notch.

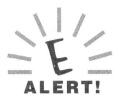

ALERT!

Whether you are just beginning or have exercised for years, you are responsible for your own health and well-being. It is always highly recommended that you speak with your doctor before beginning any new exercise program.

For the Fitness Enthusiast

Those of you who already participate in some fitness regimen or sport can also use this book. Regardless of your fitness level, you probably have a specific area of your body that troubles you and can benefit from targeted exercises. Perhaps you are a yoga lover and attend classes at a studio regularly. Or, perhaps you are one of the many new

Pilates devotees who love the results you are getting from the lengthening and strengthening aspect that makes up the base of the Pilates program. In either case, however, you just don't seem to be able to shake your conviction that your legs are "top heavy" or that the backs of your upper arms are still not ready for the prime time of summer tank tops and sleeveless T-shirts.

If you want to improve any part of your body you can use *The Everything® Body Shaping Book* and put together a quick arm-intensive or leg-intensive program as a complement to the yoga, Pilates, or any other exercise program you are already doing. By just adding on four or five quick, part-specific exercises from this book to your regular program, you can obtain results for that particular problem area within a short period of time.

Somewhere in the Middle

If you are one of the many who fall somewhere in the middle between beginner and fitness enthusiast, then body shaping will be a welcome addition to your daily routine. Let's say that you have some experience working out or participate in a sport on an irregular basis. If this is the case, creating and sticking with a body-shaping program is just what you need to incorporate physical activity into your everyday lifestyle.

You already know the benefits of regular exercise. However, your body is never sure when it is going to get a workout. Irregular exercise won't significantly affect your metabolic rate, nor will it have a great impact on the overall shape of your body. However, once you begin a body-shaping program and dedicate yourself to it, you will suddenly find yourself with a routine of regular exercise, thus creating a healthy and happy lifestyle.

What about Those Myths?

Since many of the exercises in this book use weights to add resistance to your movements, it might be a good idea to address some of the long-standing myths associated with working out with weights. Most of the exercises in this book are designed to focus on a particular body part by isolating the muscles associated with that body part. Weight is used to add resistance to develop that muscle and thereby tone and tighten not only the muscle, but also the appearance of the layer of skin over it. In the not so distant past, women were afraid to work out with weights because of the mistaken beliefs associated with the activity.

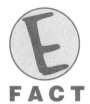

FACT

One of the reasons why building muscle with weights can change the shape of the body is because fat takes up five times as much space as muscle. Thus, if you replace the fat on your hips with the same weight in muscle, your hips will become smaller.

Myth #1

Many believe that weight training is not for women because it will make them have big bulky muscles like men. First of all, it is genetically impossible for women to build large muscles like you see on most serious male weight lifters. Women do not have enough testosterone, the hormone necessary for adding bulk to muscles. Yes, there are some professional women bodybuilders who are seriously involved in an intense and rigorous weight-training program and these women do have extraordinarily muscular bodies. In most cases these women have gone to extreme lengths to get this kind of muscle development and have applied a rigid high-protein diet to cut the amount of body fat down to almost nil levels, thereby increasing the appearance of the built muscles. However, sensible levels of weight training will not produce these kinds of extreme results.

Myth #2

The other mistaken belief is that if you start to work out with weights and are successful in building your muscles, those muscles will turn into fat if you stop. This is simply not true. Not only is it untrue, but it is also impossible. Muscle and fat are two totally separate forms of tissue. Muscle cannot all of a sudden undergo a composition change and turn into fat. The reason this myth may seem real is because once you quit training, your metabolism slows down due to inactivity. The reduction in the rate of metabolism, coupled with the likelihood that you aren't eating the best foods, allows your body to accumulate and store more fat. Also, if you stop weight training, you are no longer working those muscles. You will begin to lose that muscle you had gained. Since you are losing muscle and storing fat, it seems as though the muscle is actually turning into fat. But, as you now know, that just isn't true.

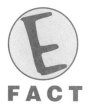

FACT

Just as muscle cannot turn into fat, neither can fat turn into muscle. When you build muscle through body shaping, you will see the muscle begin to form beneath the surface of the skin. However, you are not losing fat unless you are also eating sensibly and doing aerobic exercises.

Body Shaping versus Bodybuilding

"Body shaping" is defined in this book as a personally designed program of specifically chosen exercises with the short-term goal of changing the shape of particular body parts to reach the long-term goal of a well-proportioned and pleasingly balanced tight and toned body. This is a great deal different from the definition of "bodybuilding," which is an exercise regimen and sport in which men and women apply intensive weight-training methods to build massive amounts of bulk in the muscles and decrease the amount of body fat to an almost unnaturally low percentage, with the goal of participating in competitive bodybuilding competitions.

Since the stated goal is to "change the shape of the body," let's take a look at exactly what that means. Some of you may have picked up this book because you have one or two body parts that are displeasing to you and you want to fix them. For example, the loose skin at the back of the upper arm is a popular complaint among many people wanting to body shape. Or, perhaps you chose to buy this book because you are frustrated with the shape of your hips and thighs and think that the aerobics class you are taking is helping you lose weight but not really making your hips and thighs any smaller. If either of these describes you, then you have made a wise purchase, because this is the book for you.

While the previous are perfect examples of wanting to change the shape of a body part, some readers may want to do more than that. Perhaps your goal is to change the shape of your body, not just a specific part. Yes, overall weight loss will accomplish this to a certain extent, but after the weight comes off there is more work to do. So then, what exactly does it mean when we say "change your body shape"?

People come in many shapes and sizes and for the most part, the shape of one's body, caused by the basic bone structure, is genetically determined. You cannot do much about that. But you can change the appearance of the skin and muscle tissue that surround that basic frame, and in this book you will learn the best methods for doing just that.

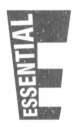

You will notice that the majority of the exercises in this body-shaping program are ones that use dumbbells or some form of weights for resistance. This is because it is generally accepted that training with weights is the fastest, most effective way to change one's body.

Weight Defines Shape

Although bone structure has a lot to do with how your body is technically "shaped," weight also plays a role in the overall shape of your body. For instance, women come in many different shapes and sizes, but there is a tendency for any weight they put on to be distributed through their body one or two basic ways. You have probably heard the expressions "pear shape" and "apple shape" used to describe certain women. Pear shapes are called such because many women tend to carry their weight in their lower bodies—in the hips, thighs, and buttocks areas. Hence, the overall impression if you look at the outline of the woman from a distance is that of a pear, thinner on top and rounder at the bottom. Women who carry weight around their abdomen generally have thinner thighs and backsides, so they are known as apple shapes because the roundness is settled in the middle.

Sometimes the body shape can change because of what is going on medically inside a woman's body. For example, some women who may have had regularly proportioned shapes as young women and adults change to having an apple shape when they start menopause. This is because hormones have a lot to do with the way the weight is distributed. As women become menopausal and have less estrogen and progesterone, they start to gain weight the way that men do: across the tummy.

We cannot control the way the weight gets distributed but we can do something about how we carry it. Of course, the best defense is not to gain the extra weight in the first place, but that is easier said than done, as most women know. However, if you have gained the few extra pounds, whether it has settled in the thighs and butt or in the belly, the best line of attack is to begin your body-shaping program!

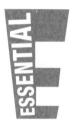

By the way, most men fall into the apple shape category. How many times have women bemoaned the fact that men always seem to have thin thighs and flat backsides? At the same time, though, most men have to deal with the classic "beer belly" or "pot belly."

The Effects of Age

Let's face it, we can't prevent ourselves from getting older, regardless of the number of age-defying products we use. But that's not to say we have to act old. Where is there a rule that says once you reach a certain age, you must cut down on your activity level, live feebly, and waste away? While this may sound absurd, it does happen. But it doesn't have to. Yes, age can make it a little more difficult to do some activities, but that doesn't mean you must become inactive. It's not likely you will be able to do the same activities at eighty that you did at twenty, so you simply have to find new activities to try! And creating a personal body-shaping regimen is a good one to include.

As we get older, we naturally lose muscle mass. If we do not have a program to replace or rebuild that muscle, there will be a gradual deterioration of muscle tissue over time. For women, this process begins in their early thirties, about the same time that their level of body fat is starting to naturally increase. Since weight training promotes muscle and tissue growth, it goes a long way to counteracting this deterioration. For those of you that are men, don't think you are in the clear. You need to rebuild muscle just as women do, or suffer a lack of strength and endurance.

Not only does physical activity promote strength, endurance, and independence, it also promotes health. Studies have shown that those who participate in some form of regular physical activity are able to delay or prevent certain diseases such as diabetes and heart disease. Physical activity also improves your mood and can stave off depression. So, to put it simply, a body-shaping program will enhance both your physical and mental well-being.

If you still aren't convinced that you need a body-shaping program, consider this statistic from the National Institute of Aging: Lack of physical activity and poor diet, taken together, are the second largest underlying cause of death in the United States. Yes, physical activity is that important. By incorporating a body-shaping program into your daily routine, you can live a longer and more satisfying life.

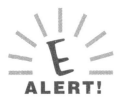

ALERT!

If you are on any kind of medication that affects your heart rate, such as blood pressure medicine, don't overexert yourself to try to reach an "ideal" pulse rate. Working yourself too hard may be detrimental to your health. As always, check with your doctor before beginning an exercise program.

What Body Shaping Cannot Do

While body shaping can do a lot for your muscle tone, overall appearance, strength, self-esteem, and mood, there are some things it cannot do. You certainly have all the reason in the world to get excited about body shaping. However, don't expect it to be the cure for all that troubles you about your body.

The Fat Attack

First and foremost, you must understand that while body shaping does burn some calories and does boost your metabolic rate, it is not going to significantly reduce your amount of body fat. Body shaping, as defined here, focuses only on strengthening your muscle tone and therefore giving shape to those muscles beneath the skin. If you want the full effect—to be able to see the newly defined and toned muscles—you will have to add an aerobic workout to the body-shaping program to reduce your amount of body fat. Since most people will want to see the results of all their hard work, an aerobic workout program has been added to this book.

Eating Sensibly

Many people are working under the assumption that once you begin a regular exercise routine, you are all of a sudden given the go-ahead to eat whatever you want. It is very important to realize that exercising does not replace the need for a sensible diet. This isn't to say that you need to go on a crash diet or not eat at all. Rather, you need to watch your intake and try to focus on consuming those foods that will provide the nutrients and vitamins you need for healthy living. The added bonus to this is that once you begin watching what you eat and concentrating on eating foods that are good for you, you will begin to lose the excess body fat, thus creating a leaner layer of muscle.

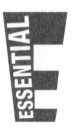

Eating sensibly will also give you more energy to carry you throughout the day. If you add this to the fact that a good diet will improve your mood, help you to reduce fat, and keep you healthy, there isn't a good argument for not eating sensibly!

Muscle Maintenance

There are several programs and so-called solutions available on the market that promise you a lean, toned body in a recordbreaking amount of time, and some of these may in fact work—for the short term.

Unfortunately, there is nothing available, including this program, that will help you take off the weight and create your ideal body shape and then maintain those results without any further work on your part.

Any exercise program is one that you must consider for the long haul. It's great to get your body into shape and feel good about yourself, but unless you can maintain a regular schedule of physical activity, those awesome results will eventually dissipate. You will lose muscle that is not regularly worked, and you will regain weight that is not kept off through exercise and diet.

Get the quick-fix idea out of your mind and concentrate instead on creating a healthy and enjoyable routine of exercise and diet to maintain for the rest of your days. Make it a part of your lifestyle. Don't worry, once it becomes routine, it will be easy to maintain. Don't let all your hard work fall by the wayside. The last thing you want to do is start all over again. Ⓔ

Chapter 3

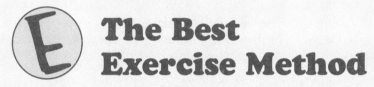

The Best Exercise Method

Personal fitness is a hot topic these days, and because of this there are several fitness programs available to you. Making a decision can be difficult when each heralds itself as the best. Don't you wish you could throw together all those "best" qualities into a fitness regimen tailored to suit your own needs? Well, now you can, and this chapter will show you how.

What Is the Best?

If you've ever spent time channel surfing late at night, you must have seen at least a few of the many infomercials touting some version of an exercise program. Whether it is an exercise machine or video for sale, all claim to help you lose weight or condition your body. You will see many different approaches and programs: aerobics, aerobics with weights, walking programs, kickboxing, Pilates, dance, yoga, power yoga, step, core training, Tae Bo, and the Bowflex, to name just a few. They all claim to be effective and probably all are.

Why "The Best" Don't Always Work

There are hundreds of different exercise programs available, all of which claim to be the "best." Perhaps you've tried out a couple, put them up on the shelf after the initial motivation began to wane, and finally decided that they simply aren't for you. If this is the case, don't worry; you certainly aren't alone. Some people have stacks of rarely used exercise videos collecting dust on the shelves or even less frequently used exercise machines and gadgets that now pose as places to hang your dirty clothes. If these methods are the best, then why don't they work for you? Because they aren't all tailored for your individual needs.

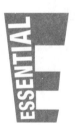

Motivation is a crucial factor in any exercise regimen. Without motivation, it is all too easy to find or make excuses to slack off. Slacking off for a day can turn into slacking off for a week, a month, and eventually quitting the program altogether.

Most people are looking for an exercise program that will fit within their busy daily lives, give them the movements they need to fix problem areas of their bodies, and will be enjoyable, even fun. While many of the "best" exercise programs mentioned will offer one or two of these incentives, most do not offer all three. The problem is that these methods are designed for the mass public, not just for you. They either do not vary the workout regimen from day to day or do not individualize the program.

This can create a lack of motivation within the individual after just a few sessions. This is where body shaping comes in to take over the lead.

Creating an Individual Workout

This book presents a program that will help you change your body, drawing from all of the previously mentioned techniques for its exercises. The focus is on you, not just the exercise program itself. You will find the information you need to target specific body parts and effect change. This book presents a mix of elements from the best of the other programs, as it puts together a workout with a specific goal in mind. The purpose of this book is to help you reshape specific body parts through the performance of resistance work with weights and support that effort with a certain amount of aerobic training and body conditioning.

You will be creating your individual workout regimen with the guidance and advice offered here. In this way, your motivation should remain at its peak level, until the exercise regimen becomes so routine that you feel the loss if you miss a day. While all the other "best" exercise programs and approaches may work well for some, this body-shaping program will work best for you. And, really now, *you* is all you should be concerned with.

Resistance Work Is Key

The core of the body-shaping program is using resistance training to reshape body parts through a series of exercises using weights. As has already been discussed, weight training is a method of building muscle strength and endurance over time through the use of resistance in progressively increasing amounts. Remember, this is not bodybuilding, which is a sport that uses weight training to build massive bulk in the muscles and reduce the amount of body fat to extremely lean proportions in order to intensify the visual effect of the musculature. This is not what we are doing in this book. This book advocates body shaping as opposed to bodybuilding: You will be using the exercises to build a shape, not to build bulk.

There are several exercise programs that are built around the theory of resistance training. This is mainly due to the simple fact that it works and produces results. The difference here is that you will learn how to build your own resistance-training program, targeting those areas of your body that you feel need improvement. Always remember that you are in control of the results that your body produces. Resistance training is a means to an end. The rest of it is up to you.

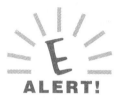

ALERT!

While building the body-shaping program is entirely up to you, please be careful to heed the advice given. Don't try to take on more than you can handle, hoping to produce faster results. This will only serve to stress or injure your muscles, thus ultimately delaying the results you wish to achieve.

In the Comfort of Your Own Home

If you belong to a gym, there are a number of machines available to you that are specific to particular body parts. The Nautilus machines at almost any gym are set up in a circuit, which, if done from beginning to end, provides a complete set of exercises for each body part. Joining a gym is a great way to kick off your fitness endeavor. However, it is not always the best way.

If you are toying with the idea of joining a gym, you must first consider the expense and time needed. The cost itself is sometimes a deterring factor. But also think about how much time it would take you to commute to and from the gym. Add this to the time of the actual workout and you could find yourself spending more time than you have available for your fitness regimen. It is essential that you be realistic in setting up your body-shaping goals. In today's fast-paced society, time is always a factor. Luckily, building your own body-shaping program within the comfort of your own home is not only possible, but also time and cost efficient.

Maintaining Concentration

Concentration is a key factor in any project you work on. Body shaping is no different. You will need to concentrate on the exercises you are performing while maintaining a focus on your goals for your body. If you haven't already guessed, this takes up a lot of mind power. The fewer distractions you have to deal with, the better. By choosing to work out in the comfort of your own home, you have the ability to create a distraction-free space in which to concentrate solely on the project at hand.

Since gyms are open to the public, it is much more difficult to keep a steady concentration with so many people around you. Granted, everyone is doing his or her own thing, but they are still there in your space and in your mind. If you happen to see someone with a body you envy, you may begin to make comparisons and lose not only concentration, but also self-esteem. Or perhaps you use another person as motivation on a secretly competitive level: "I can lift just as much as she can." While the motivation may be there, the focus on your personal goals is not. All of a sudden, the other person's goals have turned into yours.

If you can work out at a gym and put aside all distractions, focusing only on your goals and your body, then great! But if you are like most people and need quiet and personal space to maintain concentration, then body shaping at home is for you.

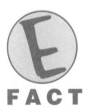

FACT

If you already belong to a gym, there's no reason why you should cancel the membership. You can still do the at-home body-shaping workout and supplement it with the benefits of a gym membership. For instance, you may want to do the weight-training portion of the workout at the gym where weights and machines are readily available, and do the aerobic portion at home.

Achieving Results

You will be provided with exercises that can all be done at home. All of the weight-bearing exercises can be done with light dumbbells that are easily purchased and handled. Since most of you do not have the availability of machines at home, this book includes a number of exercises for each body part. You can select two or three for each body part you want to work and make them part of your personal program.

After you select your body part exercises, you should decide what type of aerobic and body-conditioning exercise you want to do to supplement your weight training. While the weight training exercises do burn calories and fat, the main purpose is to build the muscle and tighten the body part. You must do the additional cardio and aerobic work to help you lose weight if losing weight is part of your overall goal. For those of you who are not overweight and just want to reshape certain body parts, the aerobic work is recommended but not as essential. You can still achieve the results you want by solely performing the weight-training exercises.

Be Creative

When you begin your body-shaping program, you will need to have the book close by in order to reread the instructions and look at the pictures. It will take only a few sessions for you to become more comfortable with the movements, and you will no longer need to follow the book so closely. After about three weeks, your movements will become fluid and natural and as you progress you can increase the amount of weight you are using by a pound or so. However, this isn't to say that the program will become boring!

Varying Your Workout

You can vary your workout and prevent it from becoming boring by adding a little creativity to your program. For example, if you are performing arm or shoulder exercises with 3- or 5-pound dumbbells, and you are familiar and comfortable with the movements, try adding a light walking step to the routine. Basically, you start with a light walking in place movement and slowly start your arm exercises after a few minutes. This not only shakes things up a bit, but also adds a whole new level to your workout!

If you choose to use a treadmill a few times a week as your method for adding aerobic work, apply some of the upper body movements you will learn here while you are in a walking mode on the treadmill. Lateral raises for the shoulders, biceps curls, shoulder raises, and back pull-backs are all examples of upper-body exercises that are easily done while on the treadmill. Of course, you will have to stop if you accelerate your treadmill to a jogging or running speed, but doing them the rest of the time on the treadmill is certainly plausible.

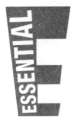

While some people prefer the quiet so they can concentrate on what they are doing, others work best in a noisier environment. You may want to try playing upbeat music while you work out. This is not only entertaining, but can also help you establish a rhythm within your routine.

Likewise, if you choose a walking program as your body-shaping supplement, you can perform your upper-body exercises while walking. While you are still a beginner, even just carrying 1-pound dumbbells while walking significantly raises the effectiveness of your walking program. Carry them at chest height, holding the dumbbells lightly in each hand, with your upper arms pressed against your body and your shoulders rolled back. As you become stronger and more comfortable with your pace and chosen distance, you can begin to do more than just carry the weights. Increase the level of your workout by performing a variety of upper-body movements such as Lateral Raises, Shoulder Presses, Dumbbell Presses on a Bench or Mat, Standing Alternate Biceps Curls, Lying Triceps Extensions, Alternate Forward Raises, Upright Rowing, and others you will learn here. (All these exercises are explained in detail in later chapters.)

Have Fun!

Suggestions like these for varying your workout will be included throughout the exercise portions of the book. For right now, all you need to know is that you have the go-ahead and encouragement to be creative with your workout. There's no reason why a workout should be dreaded. Make it fun! Your endurance and motivation are much more likely to hold out if the activity is one you look forward to and enjoy doing.

Adding Aerobic Activity

As mentioned before, you will need to supplement your weight-training exercises with some type of aerobic work and body-conditioning work. Aerobic exercise is any activity in which you exert yourself to such an extent that an increased flow of oxygen is needed to supply energy. The oxygen pours from your lungs into your bloodstream and from there your heart works to pump it into your muscles. There, the oxygen is used to break down carbohydrates, fats, and proteins into the energy your muscles need to function.

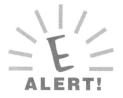

ALERT!

It is possible to have too much fun during your workout. For instance, if you particularly enjoy a specific movement, you could be tempted to do that one movement over and over, neglecting the other parts of your routine. Always maintain a focus on your goals.

This explains why aerobic exercise is good for burning calories and fat and is essential to reach any weight-loss goals. If weight loss is a part of your overall body-shaping plan, you will have to add an aerobic element to your plan. Using a treadmill or developing a regular walking program are probably the best options if you do not regularly participate in some sport such as swimming, tennis, running, racquetball, and so on. Walking is the easiest and the most accessible method to choose because you can perform it virtually anywhere, anytime, and at no cost.

Benefits of Aerobic Activity

Adding aerobic activity has other benefits in addition to providing a leaner body to show off your newly developed muscle. You will feel good, too! Regular aerobic activity has been shown to reduce symptoms of anxiety, depression, fatigue, and sleeplessness. It is a generally accepted fact that exercise elevates mood. Some people call this the athlete's "endorphin high," referring to the fact that the brain releases endorphins—chemicals that are usually associated with pleasure—during and after vigorous exercise.

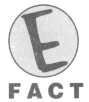

FACT

Anaerobic activity improves mood also, but for different reasons. The emotional and psychological benefits usually associated with anaerobic activities such as weight lifting have more to do with stress reduction and relaxation than the actual release of endorphins.

Before you discount the need for aerobic activity, take a look at this list of the benefits of aerobic exercise:

- Lose weight
- Reduce body fat
- Strengthen heart and lungs
- Tone muscles
- Reduce and manage stress
- Improve balance
- Sleep better at night
- Improve overall feelings of well-being and self-esteem
- Reduce high blood pressure
- Reduce and manage cholesterol
- Reduce risk of heart attack and diabetes

With all the benefits just described, you should be convinced by now to include an aerobic section to your body-shaping plan. The aerobic portion of your plan will help you burn calories and fat, display newly developed muscles to their best effect by keeping your layer of body fat very lean, reduce negative moods, and bestow an overall toned appearance.

Other Body-Conditioning Choices

Body conditioning, as used here, can be understood to mean any anaerobic activity performed for the purpose of strengthening or conditioning your muscles. Weight training is generally considered anaerobic activity. As you read further in the book, you will see that each of the chapters on individual body parts incorporates some exercises that fall into this anaerobic category.

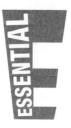

A good fitness program must be well rounded in order to have the optimum effect. Activities such as yoga and Pilates have benefits all their own and are worthy of dedicated pursuit if they are of interest to you. Further reading on these regimens is offered in Appendix B: Resources.

How Much Is Enough?

Experts differ on how much is enough and varying opinions exist on whether or not it is necessary to alternate days of weight-training exercise with aerobic exercise. Some hold the theory that you need to give your muscles a rest in between workouts so that weight-bearing exercise should only be done every other day. Another method of alternating would be to work the upper body one day and the lower body the next. Still others believe that working out every day is fine at this level of weights.

Anyone following the program in this book will not be lifting heavy enough weights to damage, tear, or even heavily stress the muscles. Therefore, you might want to apply the principle of more is better. As long as you do not push yourself past the point of comfort, and as long as you listen to what your body is telling you, it is probably safe to work out a bit each day.

You can do a full program (aerobics and weight training) three or four times a week and then on the remaining days, if you want to work out, you can do either one or the other parts of your program. A minimum of three to four times a week for each of the two parts of your program is strongly recommended though. In addition, it is important that each individual aerobics session should last a minimum of twenty minutes since any shorter than that does not give your body a chance to reach the state at which the effect starts to kick in.

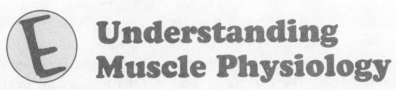

Chapter 4

Understanding Muscle Physiology

While you certainly don't need to be a health professional to participate in a body-shaping program, it does help if you can understand how your muscles work in relation to the rest of your body. The better you understand your body, the better you will be able to improve upon it. Are you ready for Muscle Physiology 101?

Types of Muscles

You know that each time you move a part of your body muscles are involved. And, of course, the joints play a part as well. But do you really know how the muscles and joints work together to make movement possible?

First of all, you need to understand that it is the joint that allows for the movement of a particular body part in a certain direction. However, it is the muscle that actually does the work to get that body part to move. Confused? Don't worry, you'll understand in a moment. Let's first look at two diagrams that show where the body's major muscles are found. You'll find these terms used again and again in this book, so it's a good idea to familiarize yourself with the locations shown here.

Now, let's move on to study the different types of muscles—skeletal, smooth, and cardiac.

Skeletal Muscles

There are more than 600 muscles covering your entire skeleton, and these are collectively called *skeletal muscles*. You are probably most familiar with the skeletal muscles—they are the muscles you will be working hard to shape within this book, in fact! Skeletal muscles are responsible for your voluntary movements—those that you consciously perform. The skeletal muscles are those in charge of producing movement, stabilizing your joints, and maintaining your posture. Because the skeletal muscles are attached to your bones, when your brain tells a skeletal muscle to move, it carries the bone along with it, thus causing your limbs to move. See, that wasn't so hard, now was it? The skeletal muscle is the most important muscle to understand for our purposes here and is discussed in more detail later in this chapter.

Smooth Muscle

Smooth muscles are involuntary muscles, meaning that your brain tells these muscles what to do without you having any conscious thought on the matter. While you may not think all too much about these muscles, they are very important to your body's inner workings. For instance, these

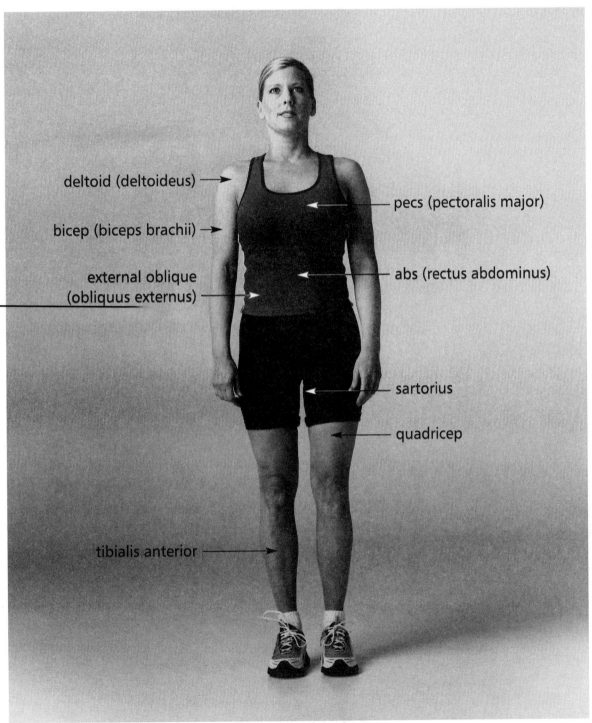

deltoid (deltoideus) →

bicep (biceps brachii) →

external oblique
(obliquus externus) →

tibialis anterior →

pecs (pectoralis major)

abs (rectus abdominus)

sartorius

quadricep

▲ Anatomy of the front

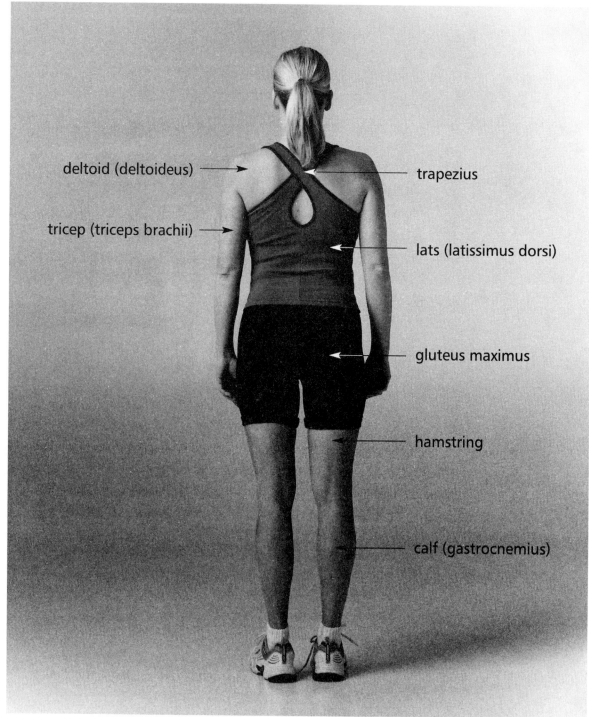

deltoid (deltoideus)

tricep (triceps brachii)

trapezius

lats (latissimus dorsi)

gluteus maximus

hamstring

calf (gastrocnemius)

▲ Anatomy of the back

muscles are found in the stomach and are used to push the food through to the intestines, thus aiding in digestion; and within the esophagus, helping food to find its way to your stomach. Smooth muscles are also found in the bladder and are responsible for holding in urine until you're ready for it to be released. Yet another location of smooth muscle is within a woman's uterus. It is through the movement of these muscles that a baby is pushed out into the world.

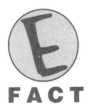

FACT

All together, your muscles make up about one-third of your total body weight. So, when you are doing an exercise program that concentrates on making the best of your muscles, it should have a sizeable influence on how you end up looking!

The previous examples are the most commonly known of the smooth muscles; however, there are even smaller and more remote smooth muscles at play within your body. For instance, smooth muscles can be found behind your eyes, helping them to remain focused. They are also found in blood vessels, helping the blood to move. They can even be found in hair follicles. While you won't be consciously working these muscles, it's important to understand that they are there, behind the scenes, playing an important role in the function of your body.

Cardiac Muscle

Cardiac muscle is the third type of muscle found in the body and as you can guess by its name, it is found in the heart. Like the smooth muscles, the cardiac muscle is also involuntary. You don't *tell* your heart to pump blood; it just does. And it's a good thing, too—can you imagine if you forgot to tell your heart to do its job?

The heart is the most important muscle in the body. It is responsible for pumping blood throughout your body every minute of every day of your life. As you know, blood is the life force flowing throughout your body. But did you know that your muscles also need blood in order to function? Well, technically, they need the oxygen that the blood carries. Oxygen enters the blood when your lungs breathe air. The harder your muscles work, the more oxygen they need and the harder the lungs and heart must work to provide it.

Contraction and Relaxation

You know that your brain tells the skeletal muscles to work, but what happens once that signal is sent? How do the muscles actually perform the action? The basic action of any muscle is *contraction*. Contraction occurs when the cells in a muscle become shorter, and tiny microscopic fibers compress and slide past each other. Relaxation occurs when the cells return to their original size. Skeletal muscles contract when they get a signal from the brain to do so. The amount of force that the muscle creates varies—the muscle can contract a little or a lot, depending on the signal that the nerve sends.

There are three different types of contractions: isometric contractions, isotonic contractions, and eccentric contractions.

Isometric Contraction

An isometric contraction is basically a "holding" contraction, meaning that no joints or bones move in the process. For example, a gluteal set is an example of an isometric contraction. As you know, the gluteals are the muscles in your buttocks. To do a gluteal set, you will squeeze the buttock together and hold for ten seconds, and then relax. You can do this exercise anywhere at any time. You will easily be able to feel the isometric contraction—you can feel the muscle tension, but you did not move a joint or limb to create the muscle movement.

Isotonic Contraction

An isotonic muscle contraction is a controlled shortening of the muscle. You will do several isotonic muscle contractions later in this book. For instance, a simple biceps curl is an exercise that produces an isotonic contraction of the biceps muscle. As the elbow bends, the muscle shortens with the isotonic muscle contraction. You can also bend the knee to produce an isotonic contraction of the hamstring muscle.

This type of contraction will be performed most frequently during your body-shaping program.

Eccentric Contraction

An eccentric contraction is the lengthening action of the muscle. Eccentric contractions occur to decelerate the body and absorb shock. For instance, the quadriceps muscle (the muscle in front of the top of the thigh) undergoes an eccentric contraction as you land on the ground after jumping off any height greater than 10 to 12 inches. Exercises or movements such as jumping, catching weighted balls, or setting down heavy objects will require eccentric contractions of some muscle groups to complete the activity.

Working the Skeletal Muscles

Skeletal muscle is the type of muscle that we can see and feel. You are exercising the skeletal muscles as you do the resistance exercises that will be outlined in this book. Some skeletal muscles attach directly to the bone and others are attached by tendons, which are like strong, tough ropes. The body's largest muscles are found in the legs, buttocks, and arms because those muscles have to move the largest bones.

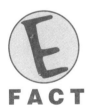

Sometimes the skeletal muscle is also called *striated muscle*, because when it is viewed under polarized light or stained with an indicator, you can see alternating stripes of light and dark coloring. Body-builders who work their physiques to extreme levels of muscle mass want to have visible striations. This condition is reached when levels of body fat are near zero and the muscle mass is highly developed.

Muscles can only pull; they cannot push. Therefore, most skeletal muscles work in pairs. When one muscle contracts, its partner on the other side relaxes. The meaning of the word "contract" in this context is literally "to get shorter." In the description of the arm muscles' movement in the next paragraph, you will learn how the muscles actually get shorter to do their work.

Let's take a look at how one muscle pair works—the biceps and triceps muscles of your arm. When you bend your elbow, the biceps muscle in your upper arm contracts and bulges, pulling the forearm bones up. The opposing muscle, the triceps, relaxes. Then, when you straighten your arm again, this muscle pair reverses its actions. This time, the triceps muscle contracts, pulling the forearm bones down, while the biceps muscle relaxes.

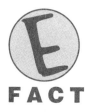

FACT

A muscle is a bundle of many cells called *fibers.* You can think of muscle fibers as long cylinders, and compared to other cells in your body, muscle fibers are quite big. They are from about 1 to 40 microns long and 10 to 100 microns in diameter. For comparison, a strand of hair is about 100 microns in diameter, and a typical cell in your body is about 10 microns in diameter.

Skeletal muscles can be further broken down into two types: fast twitch and slow twitch. You use fast-twitch muscles for short bursts of power or speed such as when sprinting or lifting heavy weights. The purpose of this type of muscle is to provide rapid movement for short periods of time. Fast-twitch muscles do not require oxygen; they use glycogen. These muscles tire quickly. Slow-twitch muscles are used for endurance activities such as long-distance running. As their name indicates, the fibers in slow-twitch muscles have a slower contraction time. Slow-twitch muscles require oxygen for power. These types of muscles are the large muscles found in the legs, thigh, trunk, back, and hips and are used for maintaining posture. These muscles do not tire as quickly.

Let's take a look at some examples of the work that muscles do in performing movements.

Muscle	Work
Biceps	Bends elbow
Triceps	Straightens elbow
Deltoid	Lifts arm away from body; swings arm while walking
Trapezius	Swings shoulder back and helps to lift arm
Lat (Latissimus dorsi)	Pulls arm back; moves shoulder
External oblique	Twists and bends body
Gluteus maximus (largest muscle)	Moves leg
Quadriceps	Straightens knee
Hamstring	Bends knee
Calf (Gastrocnemius)	Pulls heel up when you stand on tiptoe
Sartorius (longest muscle)	Bends knee and twists leg
Tibialis anterior	Bends ankle, turning sole inward

Hypertrophy and Atrophy

Do our muscles shrink when we do not use them? Do our muscles turn to fat when we stop exercising? Muscle growth is called hypertrophy (increase in muscle mass) and is caused by repeated and forceful muscular activity, such as resistance training. In muscle growth, the diameters of individual fibers increase.

Muscle atrophy occurs when a muscle is not used for a length of time or is used for only weak contractions. For instance, atrophy occurs when limbs are put into casts to help heal a broken bone. As little as one month of disuse can sometimes decrease the muscle to half the normal size. But the muscle does not "turn to fat"; it just shrinks in size.

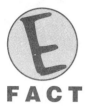

FACT

Myth: Muscle turns to fat when you stop working out with weights. This is another of the old-fashioned beliefs that has kept women away from strength training. It is a physical impossibility for muscle tissue to turn into fat. Any size you gained will be lost in time, but it will not turn to fat!

Planning an Effective Workout

Now that you know how the muscles work, you'll need to apply this knowledge to help better your body-shaping regimen. You should now understand why certain muscles respond in a particular way to certain exercises. Knowing the logic behind the exercises can sometimes give you the motivation you need to continue to incorporate that particular exercise in your program.

Keep in mind that you are shaping your body parts one by one, possibly focusing in on trouble areas. The only way you are able to reshape these parts is by strengthening and toning the muscle beneath the skin. This is why it is important for you to understand what those muscles are responding to and what makes them respond the best. Understanding how muscles work will help you target specific types of training to achieve your body-shaping goals.

Free Weights versus Machines

You've no doubt seen the many machines available to help body shape. But which is better, free weights or machines? It's best to discuss your options with a trainer, who can help you determine the best and safest way to achieve your goals.

We'll use free weights in this book, however: They're usually less expensive than machines, they're easier to store and use, and they're more practical for many people who want a full-body workout at home. Also, when you are doing your body-shaping program, you will notice that although each exercise focuses on one particular muscle or body part, the movement also affects secondary muscles. Another advantage of a free-weight program is that when you're using free weights, you are using both primary and secondary muscles, whereas the whole purpose of the machines is to isolate only one particular muscle. Another big problem people find with machines is that they provide a lot of the body stabilization. This is an important aspect of maintaining good form, but in the real world, we don't have the machine to aid us in lifting objects, pulling objects, pushing objects, or keeping our balance. It's important to learn them correctly without a machine so that it's second nature when you're performing these tasks in everyday life.

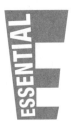

It takes fourteen tiny facial muscles to make a smile. We use other facial muscles to communicate feelings, such as raising an eyebrow or frowning. Even shaking your head or shrugging your shoulders is made possible by using your muscles.

The point is that the body-shaping program used in this book is designed so that more muscles are involved in each and every exercise. This makes the body-shaping program very efficient. If you can target three muscles in one movement versus three muscles in three movements, what would you rather do?

Utilizing Muscle Teams

Following are some examples of the muscle teams that will be used in doing your body-shaping exercises.

Exercise	Muscles Worked
Deadlifts	Glutes, thighs, lower back, and trapezius
Squats with Unweighted Bar	Glutes, quadriceps, thighs, and lower back
Bent-Over Rowing with Unweighted Bar	Lats, biceps, and trapezius

(continued)

Exercise	Muscles Worked
Alternate Forward Raises with Dumbbells	Shoulders
Dumbbell Presses and Dumbbell Chest Flyes	Chest, shoulders, and triceps
Upright Rowing	Lats, triceps
Shoulder Presses with Dumbbells	Shoulders, traps
Close-Grip Barbell Presses	Chest, triceps
Pushups	Triceps, shoulders, chest
Back Leg Kicks	Buttocks, thighs
Inner-Thigh Wide-Stance Squats	Thighs, quadriceps, lower back, buttocks
Lunges with Unweighted Bar	Quadriceps, thighs, buttocks

As you can see by the previous examples, most of the exercises in this book use both primary (primary movers) and secondary muscles. The secondary muscles being used are referred to as *stabilizers*. The stabilizers grow and increase in strength as do the prime movers, thus you achieve greater overall muscle growth.

The Proprioceptive Effect

Another benefit to training your muscles with the exercises in this book's body-shaping program is what is known as the "proprioceptive effect." Proprioceptors are small sensory tissues that help us to understand our body as it relates to the surrounding space, as well as helping us to unconsciously control our body's position. These tissues are located in and around muscle tissue.

Let's say you step off a curb without realizing it is there and battle to regain your balance. In this case, you are experiencing proprioception in action. It is something like having balance, but even more than that. Your body fights to maintain its balance even before you consciously realize something is wrong and make the conscious effort to regain your balance. This ability is a key to athletic success and is a valuable asset that you gain from doing the body-shaping exercises in this book.

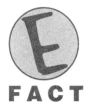

FACT

One of the strongest muscles in the body is in the jaw. The muscles that control the jaw are in your cheeks and you can feel them if you clench your teeth. The job of this muscle (called the masseter) is to open and shut your mouth firmly so your teeth can bite chunks of food.

Training Tips

Now that you have this newfound knowledge of how muscles work, you'll want to apply this knowledge to your body-shaping program. In this regard, pay close attention to the following training tips. As you go through each one, try to figure out exactly how each tip relates to your muscles and try to identify the benefits.

- Warm up thoroughly with a brisk walk or light jog, followed by stretching. Hanging from a bar loosens shoulder muscles.
- Perform exercises through the full range of motion.
- Always use good form and posture. Remember to roll back your shoulders, straighten your spine, tuck in your stomach, and unlock your elbow and knee joints.
- Bending forward or backward works the wrong muscles and can cause injury.
- Use slow, steady motions for all exercises.
- Resist gravity. Don't allow the weight to accelerate as it descends. Always lower the weights very purposefully; do not let them just drop. Always perform the second part of every movement slowly.
- Don't hold your breath. Try to breathe out during the difficult parts and in during the more relaxed phase. But most important, just breathe!

- Concentrate on the muscles that lift the weight. Visualize the muscle working. See it as you want it to be, how you want your body part to look.
- Keep your eyes open to aid balance. Watch your motion in a mirror or focus on a distant object.

We all know the importance of drinking water after your workout. But here's something you may not have thought of: Bring water along on your power walk! Fill up an empty water bottle halfway and put it in the freezer the night before. When you are ready to go on your walk, take it out and fill it the rest of the way with water. That way, the ice will melt and your water will stay cold for the duration of your walk.

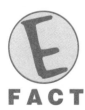

FACT

It is sometimes easy to get moving so fast while doing an exercise that the momentum is doing all the work. Maintain control of your movements and also try to maintain a steady pace in all your exercise and stretching routines.

Muscle Health

Your goal throughout this book will be to strengthen and tone the skeletal muscles to help reshape and give definition to troubled parts of your body. While you may be very dedicated to this goal, have you ever stopped to think about the health of your muscles? When your muscles get sore or begin to cramp, what do you do? Many people choose to simply ignore muscle pains, thinking "no pain, no gain." However, it's important to understand and recognize the health of your muscles. In order to do this, you're going to have to listen to what your body is telling you.

It's common for people who want to get in shape to push themselves too hard, too fast. When their muscles are fatigued and sore the next day, they feel as though they've done some good. If this describes you, try to get out of that mindset. You aren't trying to beat your body into shape, you are trying to work up an endurance and muscle strength on a gradual basis. Should you expect too much of your muscles at the beginning, fatigue, soreness, and even injury could be the end result. You don't want to do all this hard work for nothing, right?

In the next few sections, we're going to explore some of the common muscle health problems that can be the result of a strenuous workout and how to take care of these problems. You need to take care of your muscles if you want them to work for you.

Muscle Soreness

Muscle soreness is common, and in and of itself isn't necessarily a bad thing. Anytime you work a muscle that is not used to being worked, you'll feel a little soreness. It is the *degree* of soreness that you need to be aware of and watch out for. When you first begin your body-shaping regimen, you will likely feel some soreness in the muscles you worked, as they aren't used to being worked on a regular basis. In fact, if you *don't* feel those muscles you worked within the next couple of days, then you may want to take your workout up a notch. Mild muscle soreness is an indicator that you have awoken those muscles and are getting them to recognize their potential, which of course is a good thing.

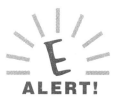

ALERT!

While most people who work out will experience mild muscle soreness, if the problem persists or gets worse, be sure to consult your doctor. You may have injured a muscle and continuing to work it will only damage the muscle even more.

On the other hand, if the muscle soreness you experience is preventing you from getting out of bed in the morning or otherwise hindering your regular daily activities, you have likely worked your muscles too hard. Unless it is injury-related soreness (which will often be accompanied by sharp pains), you should try to work the muscle slightly, perhaps by doing little stretching or simply walking around. This isn't to say you should get right back into the workout routine that caused the soreness in the first place, but you don't want to never use the muscle again either. If the soreness is too much to bear, stay off the muscle for a while and give it some rest. If the soreness is more annoying than anything else, you may want to exercise the muscle on a smaller scale than you did during the workout. For instance, you can cut the number of repetitions in half or forgo using weights.

Muscle Cramps

If you've ever disobeyed your mother and swam immediately after stuffing yourself with lots of food, you've likely suffered a muscle cramp. Muscle cramps are an involuntary contraction of the muscle that is often quite painful. The contractions are usually hard and quick, and if not relieved can create a very uncomfortable situation. Muscle cramps are common in both those who work out and those who rarely leave the couch (though the cramps would be caused by two different reasons, of course). While they are common, they aren't unavoidable.

The first line of defense against cramps is to know how they are caused. Muscle cramps are often a result of the muscle not getting enough oxygen during exercise. To combat this, start off your exercise endeavor at a slow pace and gradually work your way up to the more strenuous parts. Try to include a cardio or aerobic program within your exercise regimen as well, since these activities will help your body to pump blood more efficiently, thus getting oxygen to all those muscles that need it.

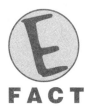

FACT

Muscle twitching, if prolonged, can sometimes cause muscle cramping. Muscle twitching occurs when a group of muscles connected to a particular neuron spontaneously contract. This usually happens without pain, but can be a great annoyance.

In addition to lack of oxygen, muscle cramping can also be caused by dehydration, stress or anxiety, certain medications, muscle fatigue, or a deficiency of calcium or magnesium in the body. If you are suffering from persistent muscle cramping, but cannot discover a cause, it is best to visit your doctor. Sometime muscle cramping can be a symptom of a major health problem. It's always best to be on the safe side. If you do suffer muscle cramps, the best thing you can do is to stretch the muscle slowly and gently. This will usually relieve the cramping; if not, talk with your doctor.

Muscle Injury

Muscle injury is often a result of pushing your body too hard, disregarding proper form, or an accidental mishap. A muscle injury, of course, is more serious in nature than mere soreness or cramping. An injury is often quite painful and accompanied by sharp pains or even numbness. You will usually know right away if you have injured a muscle, though there are types of injuries that won't alert you until a few days following the incident.

Muscle tears, sprains, and separations are examples of muscle injuries. In each case, you will want to visit your doctor for recommended care. Also, always make sure you rest the muscle for the appropriate amount of time. Don't think you can cheat and get back out on the exercise floor earlier than your doctor prescribes. If you absolutely must work out, then work around the injury, being careful to avoid stressing the injured muscle. As always, consult your doctor before working with an injury.

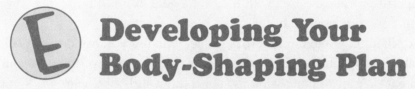

Chapter 5

Developing Your Body-Shaping Plan

It is always a good idea to create a plan for any project you are about to take on. Though you may be tempted to cut right to the exercises, you're likely to be more successful if you have a plan. This chapter will take you through the steps needed to create a body-shaping plan tailored for your needs.

Why You Need a Plan

Before you begin it is advisable to make a plan. Sure, you can just open the book in the middle, find a few exercises that work the body parts you are concerned about, do them semiregularly, and still get some results. However, you will find the results will be much more rewarding if you approach the exercises with a definite goal in mind and a specific plan on how to accomplish it.

Planning helps in all areas of life, whether you are creating a list to take with you to the grocery store or planning the wedding of your dreams. You wouldn't want to spend thousands of dollars on a house you're building without creating a plan first, would you? We plan because we take the projects we're working on seriously. Body shaping is no different. If you want to succeed, you must take the program seriously. If you take the program seriously, you must plan.

Plans are popular project management tools. Planning may be done for a variety of reasons. The next few sections will highlight some of the benefits of creating a body-shaping plan.

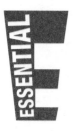

As you are reading, try to come up with some more benefits of planning as they relate to your individual situation. The more reasons you can come up with to plan, the more likely you are to take the time to do it right the first time.

Save Time

Planning saves time. In today's world, this is an appealing promise. Everyone wants more results in less time. And there's nothing wrong with that. But you must spend the time to plan in order to accomplish this.

Let's say you skip the planning stage and just open the book randomly every day and do a few exercises. While you are still doing more body shaping than you would normally do, you aren't likely to see the results you had in mind. Sure, you are working your arms, but you only manage to open that part of the book every other week. The inconsistency doesn't allow for the promotion of muscle strength.

Eventually, your frustration will either cause you to quit or go back to the beginning and create a body-shaping plan. Thus, you have ultimately wasted time using this tactic.

On the other hand, let's say you create a body-shaping plan from the get-go. You follow all the steps outlined in this chapter and are prepared each day for the exercises ahead. You needn't think about what you are going to do; you can just refer to your plan and get right to it. Obviously, you are going to see greater results faster this way. Not only are you saving yourself time, you are also saving yourself frustration.

Stay Focused

As you will soon see, part of creating a body-shaping plan is to define your goals—in other words, what you want to accomplish. By creating goals, you are giving yourself something to work toward. This will help you stay focused on the task at hand. Sure, you may have days where you'd rather not work out at all or become a little tired of particular exercises. However, having your plan close by to refer to will help you get past these obstacles. You will have your motivation right in front of you in the form of your goals. You can stay focused on the day's exercises, without having to worry what tomorrow's exercises will be.

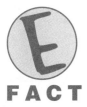

FACT

An added bonus to this is that since you have created a plan, you don't have to wonder what exercises or what body part you will be working each day. Since you have already decided this, you don't have to fumble around and try to make decisions when your mind is tired from just having worked all day or from just having woken up.

Evaluate Your Progress

One of the best reasons to plan is that you can actually see your plan being carried out. There's nothing more motivating than seeing results. If you have created a body-shaping plan, you know what you want to accomplish and can take stock along the way. You may find that you need to re-evaluate your plan from time to time. Perhaps you are seeing results faster than you expected and want to begin the next portion of your plan ahead of schedule. There's nothing wrong with making alterations to your plan. The plan is simply there to give you guidance and help you define exactly what it is that you want.

Defining Your Goals

The first step in creating your body-shaping plan is to decide exactly what it is that you want. This is probably the most important step you will make, so take your time with it. Once you are able to determine what you truly want, you will find the motivation to do what it takes to make it there. If it helps, try to think of your goals as a series of wishes that you can make come true.

Decision #1

First, think about exactly why you bought this book. What were you thinking when you saw the title "body shaping" and read the copy on the front and back covers? Most likely, you were intrigued by the promise that it is possible to "reshape" parts of your body. That is what makes this fitness book different from many of the other ones that are on the shelves—it is the promise that if you genuinely try, use the right types of exercises, perform them regularly for a period of time, and accompany your effort with a sensible diet, that you can actually change the shape of your body!

Decision #2

Okay, so you've decided that you want to reshape parts of your body. Great, you are well on your way to defining your goals. Next, think about *which* parts of your body you want to reshape. Perhaps you are happy with your thighs and legs, but want to get rid of the flab hanging off your upper arms. Or, maybe your arms are fit but you are beginning to notice a roundness developing across your middle section. Maybe you want to go for the full effect and work every part of your body. Regardless of how much or how little you want to work, be specific about those areas.

Decision #3

Once you have decided which parts of the body you want to work, then it is time to zero in on them. Let's say you want to conquer your arms. Now you need to scrutinize your arms and decide just what you want to accomplish. Are your arms too thin and need more muscular toning to give them shape? Are the backs of your arms flabby and need to be tightened up a bit? Do this for every part of the body you want to work. Remember, you can't come up with a solution until you identify the problem.

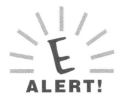

ALERT!

Don't skip this step! By zeroing in on your trouble areas now, you save time later when it comes time to exercise. This way you will be able to pinpoint which exercises will help you achieve the results you want.

Decision #4

A goal isn't a goal without an end in sight. Therefore, you need to set a time limit on achieving your goals. This doesn't mean that if you say you want toned and shapely legs within a week, you'll get it. Setting a time limit like that would only serve to frustrate you. Instead, think about how much time you have to devote to your body-shaping plan. Also, take into consideration the number of body parts you want to reshape. From here, set a rough time frame in which you expect to see results.

For instance, you may decide to devote every other day to working your legs and choose to review your results on a monthly basis. You should be able to see visible results, even if it isn't the final form you desire, within a month. Make sure the goals you set are reasonable. You may even want to allow yourself a little cushioning so that you won't get discouraged if you haven't met your goals exactly within the time period you desire.

Creating a Body-Shaping Journal

Once you have set your goals, your next step is to actually write them down. Believe it or not, your goals can seem like wishes until they hit the black and white of the page. When you write them down, all of a sudden they take on a life of their own. Here they are, staring at you, prompting you to act, willing you to succeed. Writing these goals down becomes the first tangible part of your body-shaping plan.

Start by buying or choosing a small lined notebook that will serve as your body-shaping journal. This book will become your constant companion and support as you go through the program over the next few months. The first thing you want to write down is your goals. You may choose to write these down on the inside cover, so that each time you open the notebook, they are there reminding you why you are doing all this hard work.

Of course, you can organize your journal in any way you want. For instance, you can use the book to write down your plan and your goals in great detail. Then, when you choose the exercises from the book that you want to include in your workout, you can make a list of the exercises and their corresponding page numbers. You can use it to record your progress by writing a report at the end of a specified period of time, such as after two weeks. You can keep a record of your daily exercise efforts by writing down which exercises you performed and at what level. However you choose to organize your journal, just be sure you remain consistent. There are some sample journal pages to track your progress included in Appendix C. You can use them as they are designed or adapt them to fit your own needs and program.

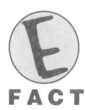

FACT

You can also use your body-shaping journal to monitor your diet. Keep information about your nutrition/diet plan, a list of your acceptable foods, snack ideas for quick reference, and even a daily food log, which you will find helpful if you are watching your diet.

The Mind as a Body-Shaping Tool

A technique that you might find useful in setting your goals and developing your journal is to use visualization exercises. If you have never used visualization exercises, you are in for a treat! Visualization is a powerful tool that you can use while you are working out. It can help move you closer to actually accomplishing your goals (this type of visualization will be discussed in a later chapter), but it can also be useful in the earlier stages as well. You can use visualization to help you further define your goals.

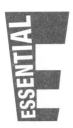

If you haven't already guessed, defining your goals is an ongoing process that needs constant evaluation and re-evaluation. Your goals may change or you may need to update your time limits. As long as you are able to keep a focus on the goals themselves, changing them around a bit isn't going to make your plan suffer.

Your Mind's Eye

Take some quiet time to visualize your perfect body. Don't try to superimpose your head over a supermodel or celebrity's body. This is cheating. Try to be as realistic as possible. Your body is going to be different from anyone else's. Shut your eyes and try to get a picture in your mind of your body. Once you can see your body as it actually is now, begin to imagine each body part separately as you would like it to be. Slowly, step by step, concentrate on each area of your body and actually see it change into the ideal. Focus on each body part and *see* the muscles develop, imagine the skin tightening over the muscles, and concentrate on holding that image in your mind's eye.

The Power of Belief

Now imagine yourself actually looking like that image you created and believe that it can actually happen. This is a type of creative daydreaming that has a real function. The more you visualize, the closer you get to actually believing you can reach that goal. The more motivated you get,

THE EVERYTHING BODY SHAPING BOOK

the harder you work and the closer you get to looking like that picture in your mind.

Just like visualizing your perfect body is a way of conditioning your mind to believe you can have it, writing down your goals is a way of making them more concrete. All this mental conditioning is a part of your body-shaping program. There is a basic psychological principle called "self-fulfilling prophecy" that is at work here. Basically, this means that the more you do that helps you believe something will actually happen, the more you condition your subconscious mind to make choices that will bring you closer to making that goal a reality. Your mind can be a powerful tool in your body-shaping program. You can program your mind to be your best ally—and when you have your mind working together with your body to accomplish your goals, you are well on your way to reaching your perfect body.

Self-Assessment

One great idea is to include a "before and after" section within your journal. In the beginning, write down your weight and your measurements. Remember, with this body-shaping program, measurements are more important than weight. Your goal is to lose (or in some cases, gain) inches. Self-assessment should be a part of your body-shaping plan. You need to be able to gauge how much you have accomplished, not only to help determine the progress of your goals, but also to serve as a form of motivation.

Measure Yourself

One method for assessing progress is to measure yourself before you start the program, and then again in regular periods. It's important that you don't do this randomly if this is the method you choose for self-assessment. Use your journal and write down specific dates on which you will measure yourself. For instance, you may want to choose the first date as exactly fourteen days from the day you start the program. The second measurement will be in another fourteen days, and so on.

If you just measure yourself randomly, it's likely you will do it too often. Measurements every other day aren't going to show you much progress and you may get discouraged. Remember, motivation is key. Use the measurements to boost your self-esteem and inspiration.

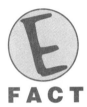

FACT

Another method to assess the changes in your body shape is to be aware of how your clothes fit. Within just a few weeks, you will notice that your clothes fit better—looser around the waist, hips, and thigh area, but tighter (in a good way!) in the shoulder, back, and chest area.

Use a Mirror

Of course, your best method for evaluating how far you have come is the mirror! Get in the habit of looking at yourself in the mirror without any clothes on. Don't just look—really study your body, all of it from head to toe. Many of you might not have ever done this! Give yourself a cold, hard once-over. This will be helpful in the beginning when you are setting your goals and developing your plan because you will really be able to identify exactly what parts of your body you want to work on. If you take a good look at your body in the beginning, later, when you look again to evaluate your progress, you will actually really be able to see how your body has changed or is changing. Another idea is to have a good friend take a Polaroid of you in a bathing suit before you start the program and then take photos of yourself in the same suit and place in the same pose at the three-week, six-week, nine-week, and twelve-week marks, and so on.

Putting the Plan into Final Form

Once you have started your journal and done your visualization exercises, the next step is to actually create the plan including your goals and the exercises you will use from the book to reach each goal. For example, if one of your goals is to get a flatter stomach, you would write that at the top of a page and list the page numbers and exercises for the abs. Another goal could be to fix the loose skin at the back of your upper arms. Write down "upper arms" at the top of the page, then all the page numbers for the exercises for the triceps. Write down what you want to accomplish with each area of your body. Be as specific as possible. The act of writing this down is another step toward reaching your goals. Every time you write down what you want, it reinforces your belief and motivation that it can actually happen.

Using all the exercises in this chapter, create a schedule that fits in with your daily life—one that you can easily adhere to. If you keep a daily planner, be sure you write down the times you are going to devote to exercising your muscles. Keep in mind, your plan may change throughout the course of your body-shaping endeavor, and that's perfectly acceptable. However, be sure you are keeping your goals in mind and are constantly working to achieve them.

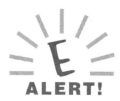

ALERT!

It's a good idea to read this book all the way through before finalizing your body-shaping plan. Later chapters will discuss issues such as the importance of warming up and nutrition. You may want to include information from these chapters within the plan.

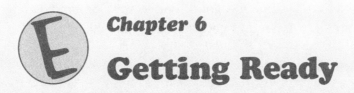

Chapter 6

Getting Ready

Now that you've committed yourself to giving this program a chance, it's time to figure out what you need to get started. Body shaping does not require a costly investment in time, exercise equipment, or space. With a minimum amount of money, you can get set up with the necessary equipment to perform the entire program. As for time, fifteen to twenty minutes a day will suffice.

Equipment You Need

The good news is that not much equipment is needed and for just a small investment, you can set yourself up at home with everything you need to work this program with success. If you do not belong to a gym, a few inexpensive dumbbells in a variety of weights, ankle weights, an unweighted bar, a treadmill or a good road to walk on, and a stable pair of sneakers are all you need to get your body into shape!

What Are Free Weights?

Free weights are metal bars with weights on both ends. These weights are either permanently attached or can be added and adjusted. Free weights include dumbbells and barbells. Dumbbells are held in one hand and can be used singly or in pairs. A barbell is a long bar that is held with both hands.

Dumbbells and barbells are called "free" weights because your body is free to determine the movement pattern that you perform when you use the weights. Machines, on the other hand, put your body into a specific position to target particular muscles. Free weights, combined with the force of gravity, simply provide resistance. You get to choose the movement.

Advantages of Free Weights

Free weights permit greater exercise variety. You have more freedom of movement. In addition to targeting specific muscle groups, as in a biceps curl, you also need to use your smaller stabilizer muscles to keep good form throughout each movement. For example, with a standing biceps curl, you need to engage your abdominal muscles, back muscles, and shoulder stabilizers for good posture. To further challenge your balance, you can perform the exercise while standing on one leg. Free weights therefore train the entire body to support a movement, rather than specific muscle groups.

Free weights are much less expensive than universal or Nautilus equipment. They are more practical for home use and require less storage space. Free weights, however, require excellent technique and knowledge of good alignment. Since positioning your body is critical to effective exercise performance, you need to pay attention to ensure that you continue to do your exercises safely and correctly.

Free weights are fixed resistance and use the force of gravity combined with the resistance of the weight. An advantage of this type of training is that it is very functional. When we use free weights, it resembles the typical challenges we face in daily living when we need to use strength. For example, doing squats with an unweighted bar (see the leg exercises in Chapter 15) will greatly strengthen the quadriceps and biceps muscles of the legs. Since correct form dictates that you should lift any weight by bending at the knees and using your leg strength instead of your back muscles, your strong leg muscles will enable you to lift any burden with ease.

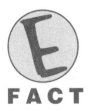

FACT

Dumbbells allow you to train each side of your body independently. This makes you aware of muscular imbalances in your body between your dominant and nondominant sides. You can use dumbbells to help equalize this strength differential for better overall muscular development.

All about Dumbbells

Dumbbells typically come in predetermined weight increments. They may be as light as 1 pound or heavier than 100 pounds, though for the purposes of this program, we will be dealing mostly with weights of under 10 pounds. Some dumbbells are coated with rubber and come in bright colors. Others are standard issue gray or black steel. "Hex head" dumbbells have hexagonal ends to prevent the weights from rolling.

One of the advantages of dumbbells is that you train each arm independently. You will immediately become aware of strength imbalances between the right and left sides of your body. Ideally, you want to improve the strength of your nondominant side. Remember, your body is only as strong as its weakest link. Using dumbbells will highlight some of these muscular imbalances and help you to address them.

Another advantage with dumbbells is that you have more freedom to alter your body position. For example, when you are doing a biceps curl, you can turn your palms in if you're holding dumbbells. This is not possible with a barbell. Therefore, you can do a greater variety of exercises with dumbbells.

You can find inexpensive weights almost anywhere. Any major department store—for example Wal-Mart, Kmart, or Sears—will have an assortment of inexpensive, handheld weights. You can choose from vinyl, rubberized, neoprene, or the old-fashioned iron ones. Choose what you like; it does not make a difference—except perhaps that the ones made of neoprene are more gentle on soft hands and come in fashionable colors! On the other hand, some devotees will not use anything other than the classic iron dumbbell—there is something invigorating and stimulating about hearing that faint clink of metal on metal when the two dumbbells lightly touch during a controlled movement.

For the beginning stages of this program, you should pick up two each of the following weights: 1-pound dumbbells, 2-pound dumbbells, and 5-pound dumbbells. As you progress, you may go back and invest in the next few sizes up (8 pounds and 10 pounds), but what is listed here should be good enough to get started. Actually, you are likely to discover that the lighter weights are preferable even though handling heavier ones might be possible and even easy. It has to do with the type of muscle being worked, and how it responds to the work, but more about that later.

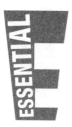

A general principle you will learn is that lighter weights with more reps tighten and tone the muscles, while heavier weights with less reps builds size and bulk. You will have a different goal with each particular muscle, and that will determine which way to go with the weight and repetitions.

Barbell or Unweighted Bar

Barbells come in fixed weights or allow for adjustment by adding weight plates. However, for the purposes of this program, you will only need an unweighted barbell (standard bar without weight plates). You will have to go to a sports store that specializes in sports equipment in order to purchase a plain bar without the weight plates that usually accompany it and are sold as a set. You just want the bar. It is also acceptable to substitute a plain broom or mop handle (without the head!).

A company called TerraStar makes a great bar called a "weight stick." It is sold along with a video that presents a strength-training program by a fitness expert named Denise Druce, and it is based on a series of movements using the bar. This weight stick, or padded bar, has padded weights on each end and the stick weighs a total of 12 pounds. It is sold with extra 1-pound weights that can be added to increase the resistance up to 14 pounds. This is a great tool for your body-shaping program, but only after you have advanced past the first six months or so because of the 12-pound weight. Beginners should stick with the unweighted bar, or even a light broomstick.

Depending on your base fitness level, you may prefer the much lighter broomstick to the unweighted bar, which usually weighs in at 10 pounds even without the plates. Both objects will work for the program outlined in this book. The advanced program presented later in Chapter 17 does have some exercises that require 5 or 10 pound plates, and this is where the TerraStar weight stick would come in handy, but the basic program requires an unweighted bar.

Ankle Weights

Ankle weights are another useful tool for your home gym weight-training workout. Ankle weights come in a variety of weights from as light as 1 pound each to as much as 5 pounds each. Some come with adjustable weight pockets so you can increase the weight as you become stronger. Beginners should start with the 1-pound weights and even advanced body shapers might not want to go beyond 3 pounds on each ankle. Ankle weights are useful for your lower body exercises. They will add resistance while you are performing your leg movements, thereby making the muscle work harder and stimulating growth.

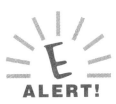
ALERT!

Under no circumstances, however, should you walk around or perform any type of aerobic exercise while wearing ankle weights. If you swing your leg without control while wearing your weights, you increase your risk of injury.

Clothing

Loose, comfortable, workout wear such as sweatpants, a good sports bra, and tank top, will be the perfect outfit to work out in. A tank top is suggested because you should be able to see your upper body muscles in the mirror for two reasons. First, seeing your muscles and body parts being worked will help you assume the correct form. You will be able to see if your shoulders are relaxed or tense, for example. Secondly, the changes in your muscles will occur so fast, you will want to see the results in the mirror as you progress.

As with every exercise regimen, good footwear is essential. Stability will be an important factor as you perform some of these moves, so a good pair of cross-training sneakers is a necessity. Your feet need to be stable as you perform many of these movements, so this is an investment you don't want to scrimp on. Good sneakers are expensive but worth their weight in gold.

Exercise Mat

Some of the exercises are performed lying down or sitting on the floor, so you will need a padded exercise mat. You can buy one in any sports or department store. Yoga mats work well and, with the popularity of yoga, are readily available in most locations. At a minimum, a large beach towel on a carpeted floor will suffice until you are able to purchase a regulation mat.

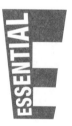

Comfort is essential while performing exercises. There isn't any reason why you should take the "no pain, no gain" approach if you can achieve the same results and be comfortable at the same time. Also, you are more likely to exercise more often if you are comfortable doing so.

Bench

The weight bench offers a number of training options with free weights. Benches are used in four positions: flat, vertical, incline, and decline. Some benches are adjustable. Others are in a fixed position.

If you are working this program from home alone and not visiting a gym, ideally, you will want to have a flat bench available. A flat bench allows you to perform both upper-and lower-body exercises. You may lie with your back on the bench or kneel with one hand and one knee on the bench. You may also use the bench for pushups, dips, and sit-ups.

For home use, a step aerobics bench with removable risers can be adapted successfully for use as a weight bench. When you purchase a step setup, it comes with a platform you stand on, along with a number of supports that can be added or taken away to raise and lower the platform. Programs such as "The Firm," a video system that uses a combination of free weights and aerobics, are sold with a small bench or platform that is adjustable and can be used as a bench during exercises that require you to use a weight bench. To use a step platform as a flat bench, use the maximum amount of risers included in the set, with an equal amount on each side. For a decline or incline effect, use an unequal amount of risers. To avoid sliding off the step, use a specially designed step mat or a towel. The mat also adds cushioning that increases comfort when lying on the step.

Develop a Routine

Everyone develops routines within their daily lives. For instance, you probably brush your teeth every morning (at least we hope so!). You've been doing this for several years, and it has become something you just naturally do without thinking about it. If you were to miss a morning, you'd probably know it. Your mouth is used to that fresh feeling and taste. To not brush your teeth would likely leave a bad taste in your mouth and give you that less-than-clean feeling that lasts all day. With time, incorporating a body-shaping routine into your daily life can be much like brushing your teeth. If your body is accustomed to exercising each morning, it's going to let you know when you miss a session. Throughout that day, you may have a lower level of energy or dampened spirits.

Your program will be more successful if you set aside the same time and place for performing it. The more set in your routine you are, the more automatic it will become. The more regular your routine, the more used to it you will become. If you then miss an exercise session, your day will feel "off" as if something is missing. Set aside a special corner of your room for your equipment, then it will be there waiting for you at all times.

Determine the Best Time

Depending on your own personal body clock, pick a time of day for your workouts that offers you the best chance of maintaining regularity and uninterrupted blocks of time. Many find that the best time is early in the morning before the routine of the day starts to get in the way. For others, after work may be the time they set aside for themselves, but this is not likely for those with children and dinners to cook! Whatever works for your personal situation, whether it be morning or evening, you should try to make it the same time each day and commit to a number of sessions each week that you will not go under. In any case, though, it should not be less than four sessions per week.

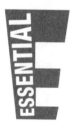

As a general rule, unless you have to be at your office very early, morning is the best time for doing your workout. Most people are fresh and ready in the morning, unlike the end of the day when it might be too easy to plead tiredness or exhaustion after a hard day at the office.

Setting Up Your Body-Shaping Area

Find an area in your house that will give you a clear 6-foot-square area that you can set up for yourself. You will need a full-length mirror so you can watch yourself work out. The area needs to be large enough to give you unrestricted range of movement and room for the mat and bench.

Keep your equipment lined up and ready so that you can get right to it. Some people find it helpful to have a CD player or radio nearby to play music. The upbeat rhythm can increase your energy and enthusiasm and help you get into the swing of it. On the other hand, some people prefer quiet so they can concentrate on perfecting their form and intensify their visualization exercises.

Keep Records of Your Workouts

Keeping records of your workouts will serve more than one purpose. Logging in your workout dates and the exact exercises performed will help keep you motivated by helping you see a record of your gains and by acting as a visible testament to your continued commitment.

The more disciplined you can be about all the tasks associated with your self-improvement routine, the better your chances of maintaining that discipline when it comes to keeping your workout schedule. If you are keeping an exact record of the dates, you will not want to see a gap the next time you go to record your progress. Likewise, if you keep a food diary in addition to the workout diary, it will help your body-shaping plan since you will not want to log in many occasions of straying from the straight and narrow. There is something uncomfortable about having to write down each piece of chocolate cake you eat!

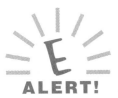
ALERT!

Don't give in to the temptation to cheat as you journal your progress. You won't gain anything by logging in extra workout sessions. Keep in mind that no one is going to see your journal. It is for your eyes (and your benefit) only.

Posture and Correct Body Position

Throughout the exercise section, you will see constant reminders to get into the correct body position. As you assume the start position for each exercise—after you place your arms and legs in the instructed positions and before you actually perform the movement—make sure that you are doing the following.

Never Lock Your Joints

Your body should be stable and steady but not rigid. Practice doing what is called "unlocking" your knees and elbows. To unlock your knees or elbows, make sure that you are not holding the joint rigid, or straight and tight. If you keep your arms almost straight but just short of locking the joint at the elbow, you will be holding your arms correctly. Ditto with the legs. Your legs should be straight but just short of locking the knee joints. One trick that will help you assume the correct position will be to actually "lock" your joints so you know what it feels like, then consciously loosen them. Then you will be in the unlocked, correct position.

Roll Your Shoulders

Before each movement, roll your shoulders back. This will help loosen and relax them, assuring that you do not use them to perform the movement. In working out with weights, it is essential to concentrate on the actual muscle being worked and not use other parts of your body to assist. Concentrating on relaxing your shoulders will prevent you from using them to compensate, or help you perform, the exercise. Rolling your shoulders back at the beginning of each exercise also aids in improving your posture.

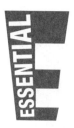

It is helpful to check yourself at the midpoint of each exercise because although you may start the exercise in the correct position, you may automatically start to tighten your shoulder muscles or use them during the exercise. Make it a habit to check yourself during the exercise as well as before you start the movement.

Don't Hold Your Breath

Without realizing it, some people tend to hold their breath while performing an exercise. This is the worst thing you can do! Remember to breathe.

Holding your breath while performing a strenuous movement can build up pressure within the chest and impede the flow of oxygenated blood to the brain. This can cause you to pass out. It can also cause momentary increases in blood pressure. Needless to say, this kind of effect can be disastrous if you are performing an exercise with a heavy weight such as a bench press.

Proper and regular breathing is important. Some experts suggest that you should breathe out during the start (exertion) phase of the movement and breathe in during the finish (relaxation) phase of the movement. That may be ideal, but the important thing to remember is to breathe regularly, in and out, during the exercise and to make sure that you do not hold your breath. If you just breathe naturally during the movement, you will be doing okay.

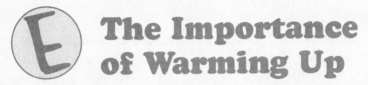

Chapter 7

The Importance of Warming Up

While you may be tempted to jump right in to the "meat" of the exercise program and skip to the exercises, don't underestimate the significance of a good warm-up. The preworkout part of your program is important for many reasons and will improve the overall quality and effectiveness of your workout.

Taking the Time to Prepare Your Body

Do not, under any circumstances, begin an exercise program before preparing your body for the workout. A good warm-up is an absolute must. Far too often people are tempted to take shortcuts in today's society. While taking shortcuts isn't always a bad thing, your body will be less than forgiving if you try to take a shortcut in body shaping by neglecting to warm up.

You might as well get used to and accept the idea that body shaping is going to take time. This isn't to say that you will have to put in hundreds of hours of work before seeing any results. It simply means that you have to look beyond the want of instant gratification. Be prepared to set aside an appropriate amount of time each day to devote to your body-shaping regimen; this includes time for warming up.

You may be thinking that you barely have time to do the body-shaping exercises themselves, much less have any time for a warm-up. Put that thought out of your head right now. If you don't have time to warm up, you don't have time to body shape. The warm-up is the most important part of your exercise routine and therefore demands time be devoted to it.

It's a pretty good bet that if the temperature were below freezing, you wouldn't jump into your car, start it up, and take off immediately. You'd start the car and let it warm up a bit. It's common sense, right? If you didn't let it warm up, chances are it would be in a mechanic's shop before long, costing you lots of money. It's the same with your body. You need to give it a little time to warm up (literally) before making it work. Otherwise, it might end up in the doctor's office before long. No one wants unnecessary doctor bills.

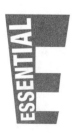

To make sure you include a warm-up in your regimen, add a warm-up program to your body-shaping plan. Write down what you plan to do each day as a warm-up exercise and assign a time limit to it. This way, you won't "forget."

The Ideal Warm-Up

An ideal warm-up would consist of five to ten minutes of light aerobic exercise and stretching movements. At the end of the warm-up, you should be perspiring lightly, your pulse rate will be moderately elevated, and you will be physically and mentally ready for the more vigorous workout to come.

A good warm-up prior to exercise fills the following functions:

- Stretching makes your muscles and joints ready to accept the stress by making them more flexible.
- Stretching the muscles allows you to achieve a wider range of motion in your weight-bearing exercises, thereby improving the quality of the exercise and the muscle development.
- It prepares you mentally for a high-energy workout.
- Stretching relieves tension and improves overall flexibility.
- Light aerobic exercise elevates your heart rate and prepares your lungs and heart for the more intense workout to come.

The actual exercises and stretches performed during the warm-up are up to you. This chapter will offer some suggestions you may want to try. If you already have your own system of warming up, by all means incorporate that into your body-shaping plan. However, keep in mind that you need to do a complete body stretch (as well as some light aerobics) for the warm-up.

Preventing Injury

You may have heard about the recent studies conducted to determine the effectiveness of stretching. These studies have concluded that there is no scientific evidence supporting the theory that stretching before exercising prevents muscle injuries. Yet, it has been drilled into our heads from the earliest days of physical education in elementary school that stretching is good. So what are you supposed to believe?

Benefits of Stretching

Well, of course you can believe anything you want to. This book advocates stretching as part of your body-shaping regimen simply because it makes sense. A warmed, flexible muscle is going to allow for a greater range of motion. A cold, unworked muscle isn't as flexible and may even be a little stiff, so it won't support that long range of motion, thus limiting the amount of work it can do. To put it simply, this program promotes results and you are more likely to get greater overall results by adding a stretching routine to your workout plan.

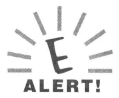

ALERT!

Don't limit yourself to stretching only those muscles you plan on working. For instance, if you plan to work only your arms one day, do not fail to stretch your legs. Your body works according to a system of cooperation; therefore, your legs will be used somewhat even though you aren't targeting them.

You have every right to argue the need for stretching. However, keep in mind that though it has not been proved that stretching prevents injury, stretching does promote flexibility. Flexibility is a desirable trait these days. Just take a look at all the Pilates and yoga programs springing up every-where. Each of these uses stretching as a foundation. Considering they are now all the rage, they must have something going for them, right?

If you aren't sold on the flexibility aspect of stretching, then consider the mental advantages. If you've ever stretched first thing in the morning after getting out of bed, you know that the stretch simply feels great. This good feeling will carry over into your body-shaping workout if the stretches are done right before working the muscles. Stretching sets you up mentally for the work to come. It will put you in the right mindset while making you feel good about it. This in itself is reason enough to stretch before working out.

The Correct Movement

Stretching may not be a proven method of preventing injury, but it can, in some cases, cause injury if you aren't mindful of your movements.

Be careful not to stretch too hard or bounce into the stretch. The saying "no pain, no gain" does not apply here! To stretch correctly, you must do it gently. Unless you stretch gently and slowly and ease into the movement, you will not receive the benefit. Stretching too far and hard may tear tiny muscle fibers and cause soreness for several days. Use smooth, gliding motions.

The correct movement for a stretch is to move gently into the position of the stretch and just as you start to approach the edge of pain, back off just enough to ease the discomfort. Then hold this position for a few seconds (preferably ten) at the top of the stretch. This principle of achieving and holding a stretch is the same as the one used in yoga.

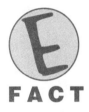

FACT

A bouncing movement causes your muscles to have a reflex reaction of contracting and this will cause your muscles to tighten up, the exact opposite of what you are trying to achieve.

Promoting Flexibility

As you already know, a good warm-up will promote flexibility in the muscles. Flexibility training is gaining a lot of attention these days as people are beginning to learn the benefits and actually feel the results of this type of workout. However, for years, fitness enthusiasts have heralded the importance of including flexibility training in fitness programs that also include cardiovascular and strength training.

While we advocate adding stretching to the warm-up portion of your workout to help you achieve faster and better results, there are several other benefits that automatically go along with flexibility. For instance, flexibility has been shown to improve a person's posture. For those of you stuck sitting in an office chair for a good portion of the day, posture is likely to be a concern. After stretching on a regular basis for a while, you will begin to notice that you sit (and stand) up straighter and don't feel the tense pressure of bad posture.

On the heels of posture is lower-back pain. Sometimes lower-back pain is caused by bad posture, while sometimes the muscles are simply holding a lot of tension. Flexibility will help to release the tension in the muscles of the back, promoting relaxation, and thus reducing the amount of lower-back pain.

Flexibility training also counteracts some of the side effects of aging. If you are older, you will likely have noticed that aging causes the joints and muscles to stiffen. Flexibility can help to ward off joint deterioration by stimulating an increase in blood and oxygen flow to the joints. The increased blood flow results in an increase of nutrients reaching the joints, which in turn promotes healthy joints.

Of course, you can't forget that flexibility also increases physical performance. The greater the range of motion you have, the more you are able to do. It's that simple. If you truly want to achieve results from body shaping, you will be sure to add a stretching segment to your body-shaping plan.

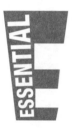

If you are interested in pursuing flexibility training beyond the warm-up component of your fitness regimen, then you may want to check out your local fitness centers. Most fitness centers offer yoga and/or Pilates classes.

Warm Up with Light Aerobics

As mentioned before, it is important to add a light aerobic exercise to your warm-up session. Ideally, aerobics should be done before stretching. These exercises will help get the blood pumping and slightly increase your body temperature, thus "warming up" your muscles for stretching. The following are two suggestions for some light aerobic exercises you can use in your warm-up.

Jogging in Place/Jumping Rope

The key to performing either of these correctly in a warm-up is to begin with a slow cadence and low knee lift with each step. Then, slowly accelerate the cadence of your steps or skips, raising your knees higher and higher until you are jogging or jumping at a fast pace at the end of the two to three minutes.

While you certainly want to increase your heart rate, you don't want to overdo it. To be physically exhausted and unable to continue the exercise program defeats the purpose of warming up. You should be perspiring lightly at the end of the light aerobic session. If you can sing without missing a beat, you haven't done enough and need to increase the intensity slightly. On the other hand, if you are unable to breathe even a word, you need to cut back. Once you get going with light aerobics, your body will tell you when you are "warmed up."

Walking/Marching

If you haven't exercised for quite a while, you may want to begin your light aerobics with walking or marching. Again, you should start off with a slow cadence, raising the knees, and work up to a faster pace. Pay close attention to what your body is telling you. You need to be stimulated, but not exhausted. A good light aerobic warm-up will prepare your body for the stretching to come. It should invigorate and energize you. Yes, you may be breathing harder than normal, but even so, you'll be ready to take on the world (or at least the body-shaping program!).

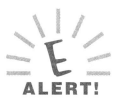

ALERT!

Do not use ankle weights while doing these light aerobics. While you may be tempted to "double-up" on benefits, you could injure your muscles in this way. Remember, the light aerobics are used to warm up your body *before* working the muscles.

Warm Up with Stretching

After you have completed two to three minutes of light aerobic exercise, you are ready to begin stretching the muscles. As an added bonus, if you repeat the stretches regularly, you will notice improvements. After months of consistent adherence to your stretching routine, you will develop greater flexibility, mobility, and an increased range of motion in your movements. Just remember to always be careful not to stretch beyond the point of comfort. However, keep in mind that the greater the range of motion, the harder your muscle is working.

Alternate Toe Touches

Alternate Toe Touches stretch the upper leg muscles, the waist, and abdominal muscles.

Start Position

Stand with your feet spread about three feet apart and keep your legs straight with your knees unlocked throughout the movement. Extend your arms directly out to the sides (parallel to the floor) and keep your arms straight throughout the movement.

Movement

Slowly bend forward and twist to the left to touch your left foot with your right hand. Return to the start position and repeat the movement to the right side. Alternate sides until you have done ten for each side.

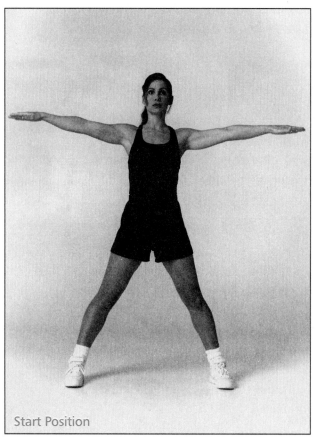

Start Position

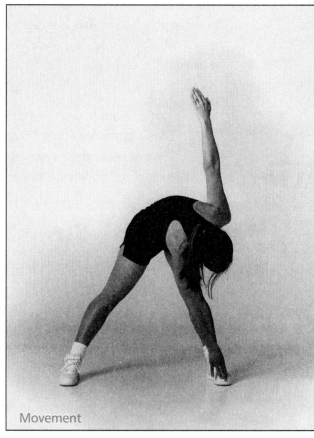

Movement

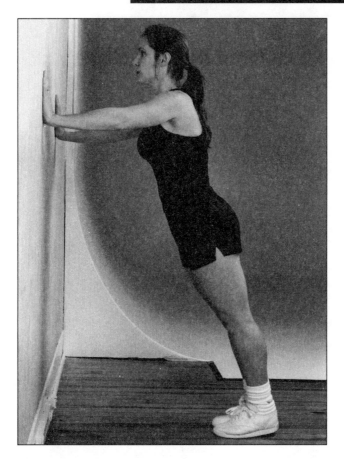

Wall Calf Stretch

This stretches the calf muscles in your lower legs.

Start Position Stand facing a wall, about 3 feet back from it. Lean forward, place your hands on the wall a bit below shoulder level, and stiffen your body.

Movement Slowly force your heels toward the floor to stretch your calf muscles. If it is too easy for you to place your heels on the floor, walk backward a few more inches and try the movement again. Hold the stretched position for fifteen to thirty seconds, then relax your calves. Repeat three or four times. If you aren't getting enough stretch out of this movement, try stretching one leg at a time.

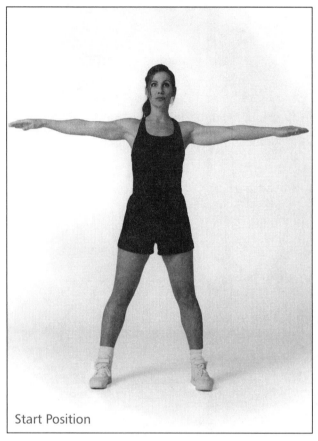

Start Position

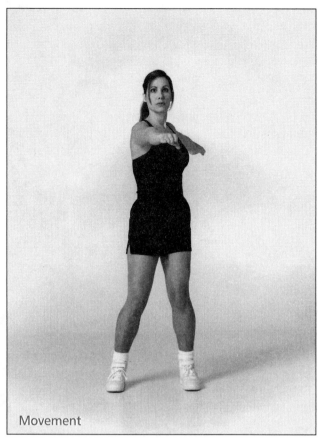

Movement

Torso Twists

▪ ▪ ▪   This works the oblique muscles at the sides of your waist.

Start Position   Stand with your feet spread about shoulder width apart. Unlock your knees and roll back your shoulders. Raise your arms to shoulder level out to the sides and parallel to the floor.

Movement   Twist your torso as far to the left as possible. Try to twist only from the waist and leave your lower body stable. Twist back as far as you can in the other direction and continue twisting back and forth until you have repeated the movement thirty to fifty times.

Quadricep Stretch

This stretch works the front muscles of the thighs (quadriceps).

Start Position

Stand facing a solid object such as a waist-high table or the top of a chair back. Place your left hand on the table to balance your body as you stretch. Bend your right leg fully and grasp your right foot behind your buttocks with your right hand.

Movement

Pull gently upward on your right foot to stretch your right thigh muscles. Hold the stretched position for fifteen to thirty seconds. Be sure to stretch your left thigh for an equal amount of time. Repeat each leg for a total of three times for each leg.

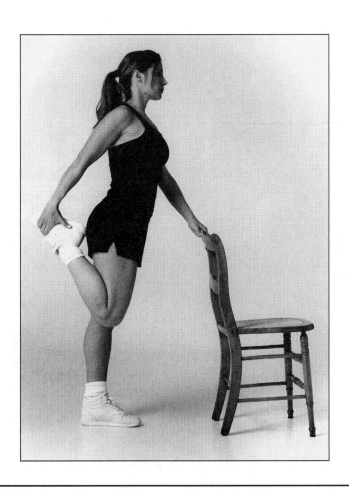

Lunging Stretch

This stretch emphasizes the front thigh muscles and hip flexors.

Start Position

Stand erect with your feet together and your hands on your hips.

Movement

Step forward 2½ to 3 feet with your left leg. Keep your right leg nearly straight throughout. Slowly bend your left leg as fully as you can and lower your hips as close to the floor as possible. Your knee should be in line with your ankle. Hold for fifteen to thirty seconds and return to the start position. Reverse position for the other leg and do an equal amount of stretches for each side, three times each.

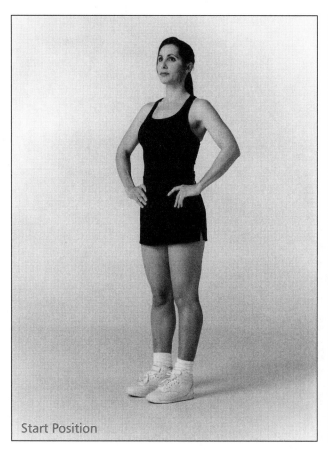

Start Position

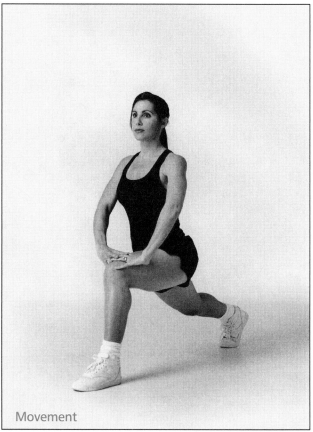

Movement

Start Position

Movement

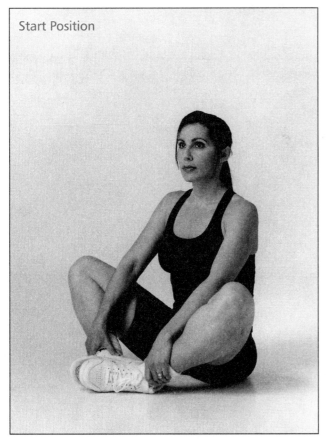
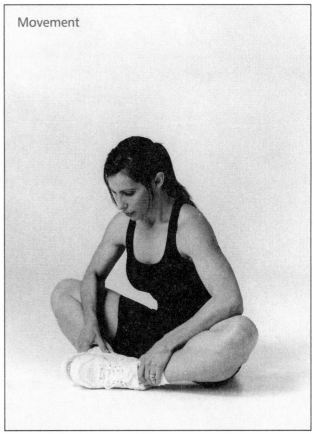

Inner-Thigh Stretch

∎ ∎ ∎   This stretches the muscles on the inside of your thigh (adductors).

Start Position   Sit on the floor with your legs bent and the soles of your feet against each other. Pull your feet as close to your hips as possible.

Movement   Push down gently on your knees to stretch the inner-thigh muscles. Hold down lightly for fifteen to thirty seconds and repeat three times. If you are feeling any discomfort in doing this stretch, try this alternative: Sit on the floor with your legs outstretched straight, relaxed, and apart. Reach forward towards your toes until you feel a light to moderate tension. Hold for fifteen to thirty seconds.

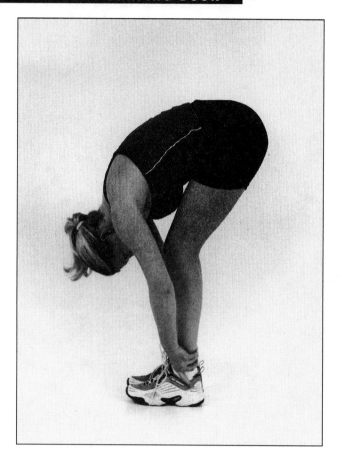

Hamstring Stretch

- - - This movement stretches the hamstrings, or the backs of your thighs.

Start Position Stand up straight with your feet together and knees unlocked.

Movement Allowing for only a slight bend in the knees, slowly bend forward until you feel a light to moderate stretch in the hamstrings. Hold for fifteen to thirty seconds.

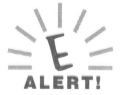

Be careful not to bounce while doing any of these stretches.
All stretches should be performed in a static position.

Side-Bend Stretch

This works the oblique muscles at the sides of the waist.

Start Position

Stand erect with your feet set apart just slightly wider than your shoulders. Place your right hand on your right thigh and extend the left arm directly above your head. Keep your legs straight but your knees unlocked.

Movement

Bend directly to the right side as far as is comfortable and hold for fifteen to thirty seconds. When you finish bending to the right, switch arms placing your left hand on your left thigh for support and bend to the left for an equal amount of time. Repeat each side three or four times. An alternative would be to perform this stretch in a sitting position with your legs apart. Stretch one arm up and over while the other hand is on the floor for support.

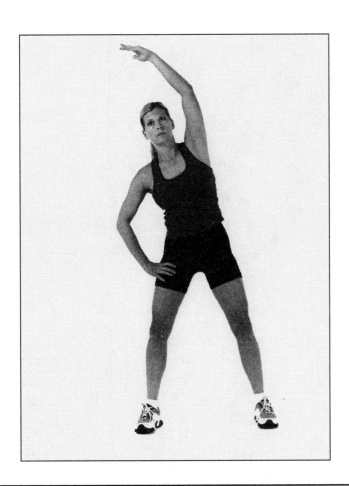

Lower Back Stretch

This stretches the muscles of the lower back.

Start Position

Stand and gently squat in a semiseated position, making sure that your bent knees do not go beyond your toes. Place your hands facing in on your mid-thighs.

Movement

Tuck in your abs and round your back while exhaling. Hold for fifteen to thirty seconds. Inhale as you release your back.

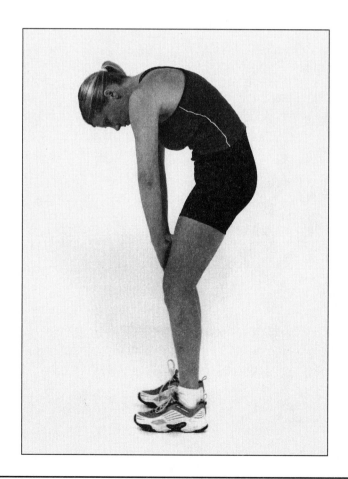

Start Position

Movement

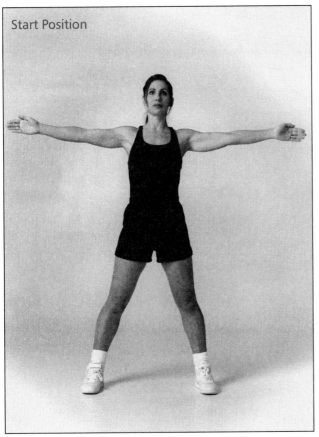

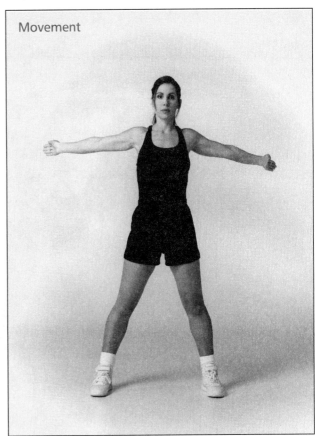

Chest Stretch

• • ■ This stretches the muscles of the chest.

Start Position   Stand with your feet slightly wider than shoulder width apart. Raise your arms out to the sides, parallel with the ground. Your palms should be facing the front.

Movement   Slowly move your arms backward until you feel the stretch across your chest. Hold this position for fifteen to thirty seconds and relax. Repeat the movement once more. An alternative would be to stand in a doorway with your arms parallel to the floor and palms facing forward. Step into the doorway until you feel a light to moderate stretch across the chest and biceps.

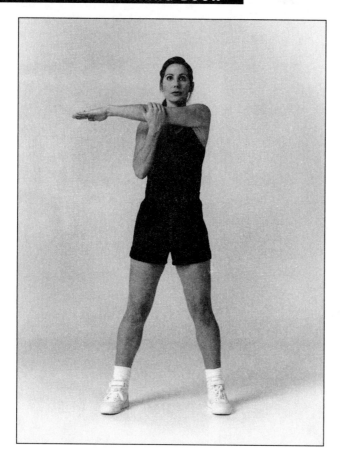

Shoulder Stretch

▪ ▪ ▪   This movement stretches the muscles of the shoulders.

Start Position   Stand with your feet shoulder-width apart and your knees slightly bent. Position your left arm across your chest, parallel with the ground.

Movement   Using your right hand, pull the left arm in closer to your chest. Hold this position for fifteen to thirty seconds and relax. Repeat with the other arm. You should feel the stretch in the shoulder.

Upper Back Stretch

This stretches the upper back, an area that is often neglected during stretching routines.

Start Position

Stand with your feet shoulder-width apart and your knees slightly bent. Bring your hands together just below your waist and interlock the fingers.

Movement

Movement: Bring your arms out straight in front of you with the palms facing front. Stretch your arms as far as you can in front of you. (You will know you are doing the movement correctly when you feel the stretch between your shoulder blades.) Hold for fifteen to thirty seconds and relax. Repeat this movement two to three times.

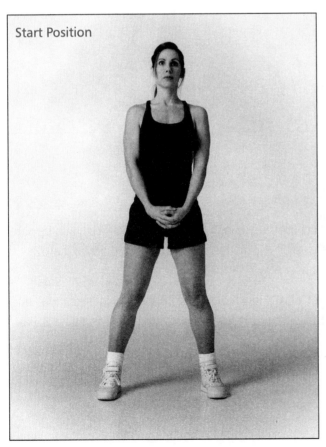

Start Position

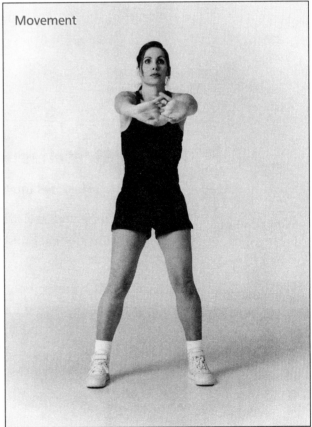

Movement

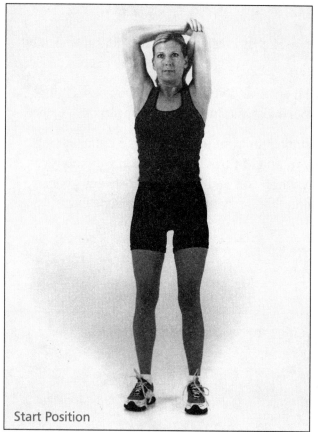

Start Position

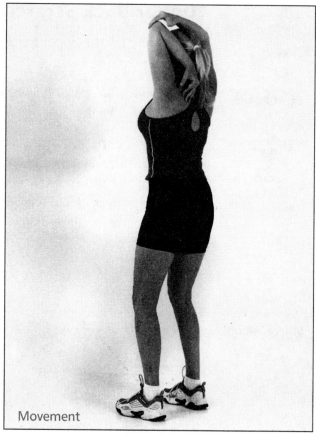

Movement

Triceps Stretches

■ ■ ■ This movement stretches the triceps muscles.

Start Position Standing up, raise your left arm straight up over your head and keep your upper arm close to your head. Bend the elbow and let the hand come down below and behind your head.

Movement Place your right hand on your left elbow and slowly pull down until you feel the stretch in your tricep. Hold for fifteen to thirty seconds. Switch arms and repeat the movement for the opposite arm.

Neck Stretches

The neck is quite fragile, so you want to stretch it gently.

First Stretch

Stretch your right ear up to the sky, lengthening along the line of your neck. Do not contract the side opposite to the stretch by trying to get the ear to the shoulder, because this can compress your neck!

Second Stretch

Hang the weight of your left arm on your right shoulder and stretch the right side again. Repeat on the left side.

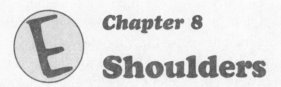

Chapter 8

Shoulders

Shoulder work will result in fast and dramatic changes, and this will be rewarding for you both psychologically and visually. Strong shoulders can impact the overall visual effect of a person's shape almost more than any other single muscle. So, are you ready to begin strengthening the shoulders?

Reasons for Sculpting the Shoulders

When the shoulder muscles are developed, the visual effect is striking. The top part of the shoulder gets definite "lines" and indents form, showing the development. Also, the overall broadness contributes to a V shape, giving the illusion of a smaller waist.

If you have trouble with maintaining the motivation needed to complete your body-shaping plan, then you will likely want to add shoulder work to your regimen. Because the shoulders typically don't bear the amount of fat that other areas are known for (such as the abs and thighs), the results of your efforts can be seen rather quickly. The visual effects can do a lot for your motivation level. Everyone likes to see results, and those results will spur you into action, providing you with the determination to achieve those same results on other areas of your body.

Toning and sculpting the shoulders also adds to the overall strength of your arms. Even if you haven't quite achieved the muscular arms you crave, strong shoulders can make the arms seem stronger than they are. On the flip side of that, if you have strong arms but weak shoulders, the effect can be a little jarring. You need to provide proportion to the areas of your body. One area affects the look of another.

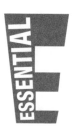

The strength of your shoulders affects the amount of work your arms can do. The shoulders bear the responsibility of your arms' movement. Thus, when you limit the strength your shoulders can handle, you are also limiting the strength your arms can handle.

Anatomy of the Shoulders

The anatomy of the shoulders shows us that there are three distinct parts to the muscle group. Like the triceps, this muscle has three heads: the side deltoid, the rear or posterior deltoid, and the front or anterior deltoid. All three areas need to be developed in order to produce strong, well-rounded shoulders.

Developing the side deltoid adds width. This is the part of the shoulder that when developed, most dramatically affects appearance. If you want to get an idea of how much of a difference adding width will make, put on a tight T-shirt and then put a folded sock underneath on the outer part of each of your shoulders and look in the mirror. Just that inch more on either side makes a dramatic difference!

Developing the rear deltoid will greatly affect your overall look by improving your posterior appearance, or view from behind. Well-developed rear deltoids prevent you from looking "round-shouldered" and aid in better posture.

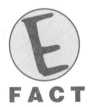

FACT

The four muscles that make up the rotator cuff are the subscapularis, the supraspinatus, the infraspinatus, and the teres minor. The supraspinatus is the most commonly injured muscle of the rotator cuff and is therefore considered to be the weak link.

The front deltoids are important because they tie in with the upper pectorals, or chest, muscles. Well-developed front deltoids help your appearance by rounding out the shoulder and increasing the impression of width from the front.

Another set of muscles in the shoulder is called the rotator cuff. The rotator cuff is composed of a group of four muscles that work together to move your shoulder joint. For instance, when you lift your arm up over your head, you are utilizing these muscles. The rotator cuff is located directly beneath the deltoid muscle.

Exercises for the Shoulders

If you want to wear tank tops or backless dresses with pride, then you need to work those shoulders! As for the men, sculpting the shoulders adds definition to the upper part of your body, giving you that look of virility. Shaping the shoulders is easy and fun. You will likely see results rather quickly and begin to show off those sexy shoulders in just a few weeks' time. Keep a visual in mind as you do these exercises of how you would like your shoulders to look. It will help you to achieve the results you want. The exercises provided here will give you a full program for the shoulders and have been selected so that all parts of the muscles are worked, particularly the deltoids, or "delts."

Do's and Don'ts

Before beginning the exercises, take a few moments to review some general exercise do's and don'ts:

- **Warm up.** Do light aerobics and stretch before working out to prepare your body for the exercises to come.
- **Follow a routine.** Set aside a quiet place and a regular time for your workout.
- **Take it easy.** Don't overtrain any body part. Avoid injury by "listening" to your body.
- **Visualize.** Concentrate on the muscle being worked—"see it" contract and tighten in your mind's eye.
- **Breathe.** Continue with regular breathing as you work out. Avoid the tendency to hold your breath as you exert yourself.

The shoulders can be a very stubborn body part to shape and strengthen—if you don't know what you are doing. It is important that you always follow the specific directions (as well as the general guidelines) when exercising any body part, and the shoulders aren't an exception to this rule. While the exercises offered here can produce quick and optimum results, they can only do so when performed correctly. Should you position your body in even the slightest variation of form, you may not get the results you want, or even worse, you could injure yourself. Watch yourself in the mirror and pay close attention to the alignment and form of your body as you do these exercises, and you can show off those lean and shapely shoulders in no time.

Lateral Raises with Dumbbells

■ ■ ■ This is an excellent exercise for the shoulders. It develops, strengthens, and shapes all the parts of the deltoid muscle.

Start Position
Hold a light dumbbell in each hand. Position your arms in front of your body with your elbows unlocked and your palms facing each other. Roll your shoulders back, unlock your knees, tuck in your stomach, and breathe slowly.

Movement
Slowly raise both dumbbells out to your sides at the same time, bringing the weights up to chest level. As you raise your arms, keep your elbows unlocked and your palms facing down. Slowly lower the weights back to the original position. Repeat ten times. Do three sets of ten repetitions.

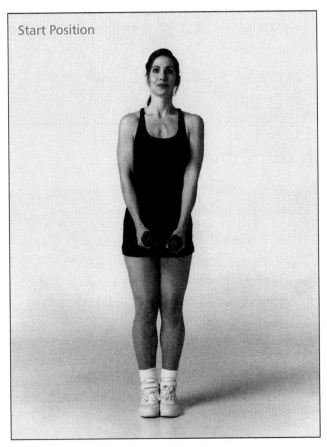

Start Position

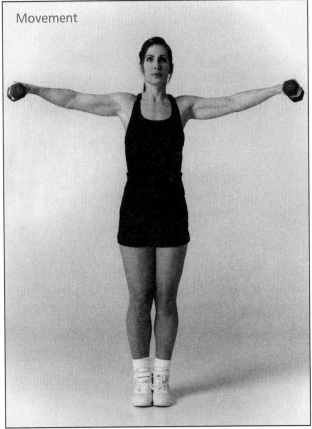

Movement

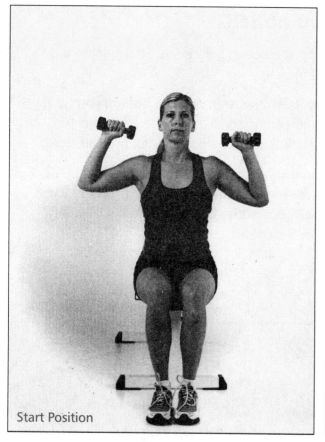

Start Position

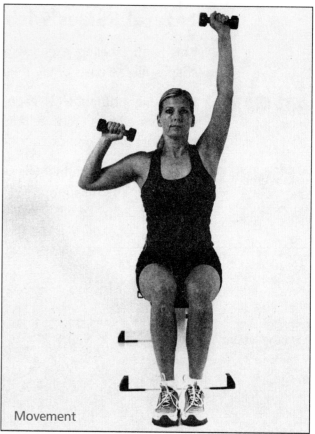

Movement

Shoulder Presses with Dumbbells

■ ■ ■ This exercise puts primary emphasis on the deltoids, but also has secondary benefits for the trapezius muscles and the triceps muscles.

Start Position You can do these standing but seated will take the pressure off the lower back. Sit on a bench or chair without a back and place your feet flat on the floor. With a light dumbbell in each hand, place your hands at ear level, elbows bent with your forearms at a right angle to your upper arm. Roll your shoulders back and tuck in your stomach.

Movement Slowly extend one arm upward until your arm is straight. Return your arm to the original position. Repeat ten times. Switch arms and repeat the exercise ten times. Do three sets of ten repetitions for each arm.

Alternate Front Raises with Dumbbells

This exercise works the front part of the shoulder muscle and places secondary emphasis on the upper pectorals, or chest.

Start Position

Hold a light dumbbell in each hand and stand with your feet slightly apart, with your arms at rest at your sides. Unlock your knees, tuck in your stomach, and roll your shoulders back.

Movement

Slowly raise your right arm forward, lifting it straight up in front of you, until it is slightly above chest height. The dumbbell should be grasped lightly with your palm facing the floor for the entire movement. Slowly lower your arm back to the original resting position at your side. Repeat the movement with your left arm. Do ten repetitions with each arm, alternating one after another. Do three sets of twenty repetitions (ten for each arm).

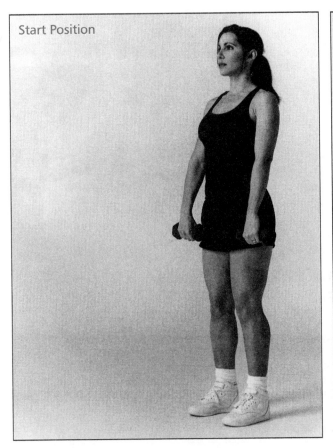
Start Position

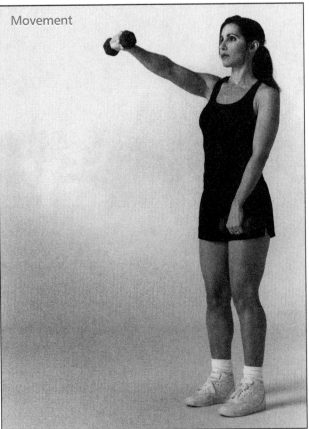
Movement

Bent-Over Flyes

■ ■ ■ This exercise develops the rear part of the shoulder muscles with secondary benefit to the back muscles, particularly the latissimi dorsi, or "lats," and the middle trapezius.

Start Position

Sit on the long end of a weight bench with your feet slightly apart and flat on the floor. Hold a 3 to 5 pound dumbbell in each hand. Bend over at the waist, keeping your upper body parallel to the floor. Extend your arms toward the ground and hold the weights next to your calves, with your elbows slightly bent and the palms of your hands facing each other. Keep your neck in a neutral position.

Movement

Slowly raise each dumbbell out to the sides and squeeze your shoulder blades together, making sure to keep your elbows slightly bent during the movement. Hold in the raised position for a second before slowly lowering the dumbbells to the original start position. Repeat this movement for three sets of ten repetitions.

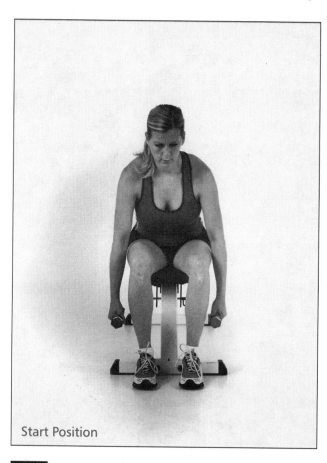

Start Position

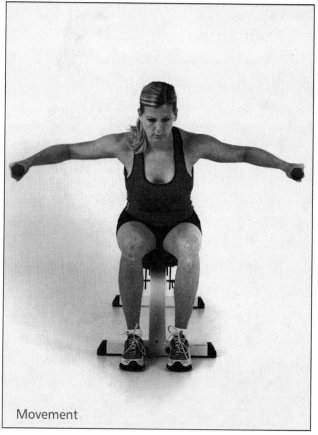

Movement

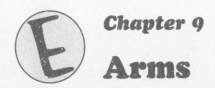

Chapter 9

Arms

This chapter is going to focus on the arms. You will learn all you need to know about the biceps, triceps, and the forearm. By following the exercises outlined in this chapter, you will be well on your way to toning and sculpting those muscles for strong and beautiful arms. Are you ready to begin?

Anatomy of the Arms

Since the basic premise of this program is that you can reshape different parts of your body by working on the muscles underneath, an understanding of what those muscles look like will aid in the visualization process that is so important when you perform a movement. There are three major muscle groups in the arms: the biceps, triceps, and the forearm.

The Biceps

The biceps is the muscle that bulges in the upper arm between the shoulder and the crook of the elbow. It is a two-headed muscle with a long head and a short head, and with maximum development you can actually see the split between the two heads. In a close-up view of an arm with a fully developed biceps muscle, the bulging and rounded part of the muscle looks like a little hill sitting on top of a bigger hill. The basic function of this muscle is to lift and curl the arm and to pronate (twist downward) the wrist.

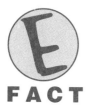

FACT

If you're a woman, you do not need to be afraid of building huge muscles and looking like Arnold Schwarzenegger! Women do not have the testosterone needed to build huge muscle mass as men do. If you see a picture of a woman with a body like Schwarzenegger, chances are great that she had to take steroids (artificial testosterone) to get muscles of that size.

The Triceps

The triceps muscle is in the back of the upper arm located directly opposite the biceps. The Latin word *triceps* means "three-headed" and comes from the fact that the muscle has three heads: an inner, outer, and middle head. The triceps muscle is used when you extend the arm and the forearm and when you bring the arm in toward your body.

For people who want to firm up the back of the arms, triceps exercises are the ones you want to include. Most women will recognize the need for working the triceps muscle—just think of how many women you have heard complain about the skin that "hangs" from the back of the upper arm when they wave goodbye! Since these muscles aren't challenged a lot in daily activities, most people tend to have weak triceps.

It is essential to perform triceps exercises with perfect form. Doing triceps movements incorrectly can put strain on the elbow joint and cause elbow injuries. The best way to avoid this is to perform the movements slowly and constantly check your form. Make sure your arms are in the correct position in the start and finish phases of the movement and visualize the triceps muscle working so you are sure to put the stress on the right part of the arm and not your neck, shoulders, or elbow.

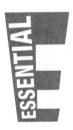

Always remember to train your triceps when you train your biceps. The synergistic work of the biceps and triceps is a perfect example of how our muscles work together. When your biceps contract, your elbow bends and your triceps stretch. When you contract your triceps, your arm straightens out and your biceps stretch. It is important to maintain balanced muscle development so one group of muscles does not overpower the other.

The Forearm

The forearm is a group of muscles (including the flexors and the extensors) on the outside and inside of the lower arm that control the actions of the hand and wrist. The basic function of the forearm flexor muscles is to curl the palm down and forward. The basic function of the forearm extensor muscles is to curl the knuckles back and up.

The muscles in your forearm control your wrist and hand actions. Strengthening these muscles are not likely to win beauty points, but you will score big in the functional-fitness column. Every time you bend your wrist or make circles with your hands, you use your forearm muscles. In addition to controlling movements, your forearm muscles act as important stabilizers for your wrists. The strength of your forearms also determines your grip strength.

You may wonder about the need for a section on forearms. While it is true that the forearms are used to some extent in many other exercises and get developed in a secondary way, it is still important to perform at least one or two exercises directly focused on the forearm muscle. If you do not neglect this part of your arm, you will be rewarded with a strong, toned arm that is well balanced instead of an arm that is "top-heavy" with a developed bicep and tricep and a thin, underdeveloped forearm.

Strengthening your forearms will not only help you to perform activities that use your hands but it will also help you do more exercises that require wrist stabilization. Strong wrists also help prevent injuries. For instance, golfer's elbow or tennis elbow can be avoided by strengthening the forearm muscles. Strong wrists can prevent injuries associated with tendonitis, since strong muscles prevent excessive strain on joints.

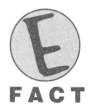

FACT

It is a generally accepted fact that the forearms, along with the calves, are the toughest muscles to develop. Using the training method of "pyramiding" (increasing the reps and weight with each set) is an effective way to get the muscle to respond.

Sculpting the Biceps

Some of you may balk at the thought of exercises designed specifically to increase the size of the biceps. If there is any muscle that is associated with the now-dated perception of weight training as being for males only, it is the biceps muscle. Just the word invokes a picture of Popeye sprouting his bursting biceps muscle immediately after eating his spinach. Images of tattoo-encrusted arm wrestlers flexing their biceps as they challenge each other add to our reluctance to work this muscle. Let's try to substitute some more desirable images for these in order to help you visualize how strong biceps muscles will improve the overall appearance of your arms, and therefore your body shape.

Think of some of the women we see daily in our popular culture who have strong, sexy arms: Have you seen Jennifer Garner on *Alias*? How about Britney Spears or Christina Aguilera for the younger set? Angelina Jolie in *Tomb Raider*? Jennifer Aniston on *Friends*? All of these popular celebrities have noticeable well-developed muscles, which are constantly being shown off with sleeveless T-shirts, strapless gowns, or a number of athletic stunts, as is the case with Sarah Michelle Gellar in *Buffy the Vampire Slayer*. Madonna is a more extreme example but bears honorable mention here for being one of the first female stars to obtain her shape by using weight training and showing off her muscles with body-baring outfits. Each of these women has arms that announce the fact that they have used weights to shape them. None of them have bulging, ugly biceps—instead they have toned, shapely, strong arms, and a small, tight, shapely mound where the biceps muscle is.

If you are convinced that strong arms look good, working the biceps muscle is of prime importance in obtaining this goal. Here are some exercises to get you there!

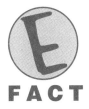

FACT

Don't forget that you are burning calories while you are performing exercises with weights! In addition to the calories burned performing the work, adding muscle will help you metabolize more calories daily because muscle burns about forty-five more calories per pound than fat tissue burns.

Do's and Don'ts

Before beginning the exercises, take a few moments to review some general exercise do's and don'ts:

- **Warm up.** Do light aerobics and stretch before working out to prepare your body for the exercises to come.
- **Follow a routine.** Set aside a quiet place and a regular time for your workout.
- **Take it easy.** Don't overtrain any body part. Avoid injury by "listening" to your body.
- **Visualize.** Concentrate on the muscle being worked—"see it" contract and tighten in your mind's eye.
- **Breathe.** Continue with regular breathing as you work out. Avoid the tendency to hold your breath as you exert yourself.

Standing Alternate Biceps Curls with Dumbbells

This exercise strengthens and shapes the biceps muscles of the arms and places secondary stress on the flexor muscles of the forearms.

Start Position Stand with your feet about shoulder-width apart. Roll back your shoulders and unlock your joints. Gently hold a 5-pound dumbbell in each hand with your palms facing your body. Relax your shoulders, unlock your knees, tighten your abdominals, and keep neutral wrists.

Movement Turn your wrist so that your palm is facing outward. Bend your elbow and slowly raise the weight up to your shoulder height. Concentrate on tightening your biceps muscle as you raise the weight while keeping your elbow at your side. Do not rock your body or excessively arch your back. Do three sets of ten repetitions for each arm.

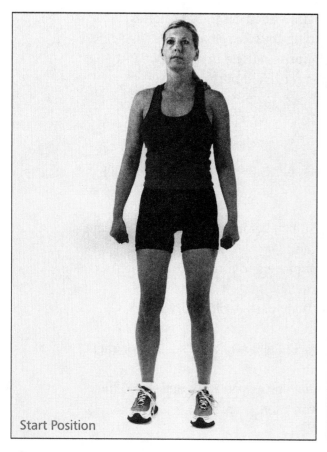

Start Position

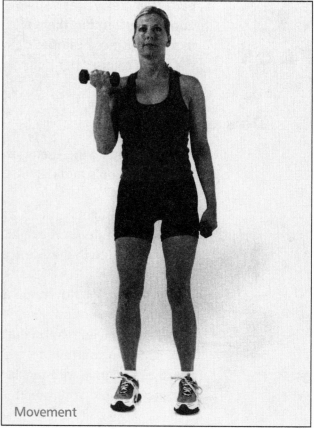

Movement

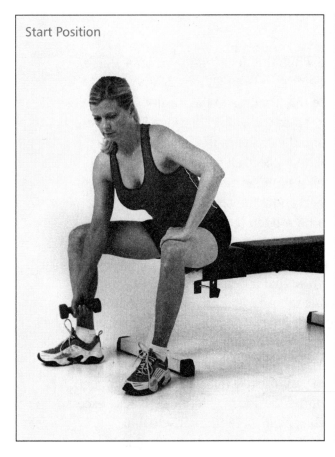

Start Position

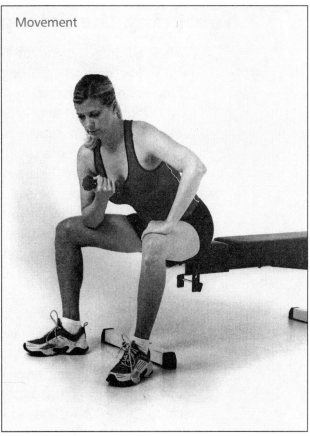

Movement

Seated Concentration Curls

▪ ▪ ▪ This exercise is great for isolating the biceps muscle and adding development and shape to the arm.

Start Position Sit on a flat bench with a wide stance and your feet flat on the floor. Gently hold a 5-pound dumbbell in one hand. Lean forward and stabilize your upper arm against your inner thigh. Your palm is facing your other leg and your abs are tucked in.

Movement Bend your elbow and lift the weight as high as is comfortable toward your shoulder. Concentrate on tightening your biceps muscle as you raise the weight. Pause momentarily at the top of the movement and squeeze your biceps. Lower slowly. Do three sets of ten repetitions for each arm.

Sculpting the Triceps

Almost all women dread the time when the decision to put on a sleeveless shirt will become an agonizing dilemma. It is an all too common complaint of women that they lose the firmness in their arms as they age and no amount of dieting or weight loss will get rid of those loose pockets of skin that starts to develop around the backs of the upper arms.

This is one of those problems that affect all women, regardless of their weight situation. Even women who have never had a problem with being overweight can be concerned about the shape of their arms as they age. Moreover, most women have been led to believe that there is nothing that can be done about this problem. Though it may be true that success is achievable to a greater or lesser degree depending on the severity of the problem, it is also true that a dedicated regimen of body shaping using weights and targeting the problem area will result in a tighter, shapelier, more toned upper arm!

The triceps is the muscle that determines the shape of the back of the upper arm—the better shape your triceps are in, the better shape your upper arms will be in. Developing your triceps will create a firm upper arm. By building up the muscle under the loose skin, there is less excess skin to "hang." A well-developed biceps muscle (the muscle that determines the shape of the front of the upper arm) will provide balance.

Because the triceps is a larger muscle mass than the biceps, it needs more training. While many upper-body exercises involve use of the triceps, there are some that isolate the particular muscle and put the stress directly on the triceps muscle. These are the ones to select when spot training, or part sculpting, since they target the area of choice.

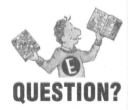

QUESTION?

Will using weights make my arms big and bulky?
No, you must remember that women do not have the genetic potential to develop large muscles because of the lack of testosterone. Any gains you make in muscle size will instead be seen as added feminine "curves"!

Dumbbell Kick-Backs

▪ ▪ ▪   This exercise strengthens the triceps muscle and the elbow and shoulder joints.

Start Position

Holding a light dumbbell in your left hand, stabilize yourself by placing your right hand and right knee on a bench, keeping your right elbow unlocked. Keep your left foot flat on the floor and your knee unlocked. Maintain a neutral neck position and tuck in your abs. Lean over so your back is parallel to the floor. Hold the upper part of your left arm firmly against your body and leave it there for the entire movement of the exercise. The lower part of your arm holding the dumbbell is perpendicular to the floor.

Movement

Slowly extend your lower arm backwards until your arm is straight out to the back, remembering to keep the upper part of your arm motionless and pressed against your body. Hold for five seconds. Slowly bend the lower arm back to its original position. Do three sets of ten repetitions for each arm.

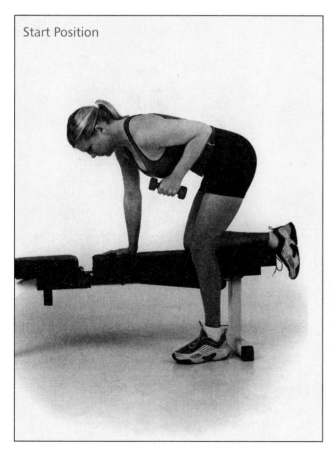

Start Position

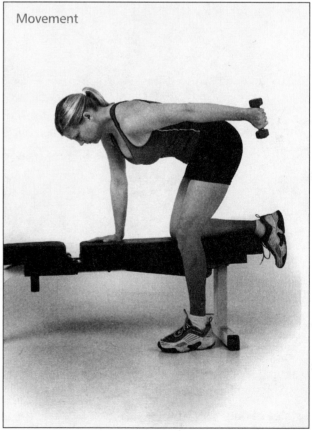

Movement

One-Arm Dumbbell Extensions

▪ ▪ ▪ This exercise strengthens and isolates the triceps muscle. If the movement is difficult at first, support your elbow with your nonworking hand.

Start Position Stand with your feet shoulder-width apart. Unlock your knees, roll your shoulders back, and keep your spine straight and abs tucked in. Hold a light dumbbell in your left hand (palm facing inward) and raise your arm straight up, keeping your upper arm close to your ear.

Movement Slowly bend your elbow, lowering the dumbbell just past a 90 degree angle until light stress is felt in the tricep. Slowly raise the weight to its starting position, extending the elbow. Do three sets of ten repetitions for each arm. Remember to listen to your body. If you start to feel elbow pain or discomfort in the joint, modify how far you bend your elbow depending upon your level of comfort.

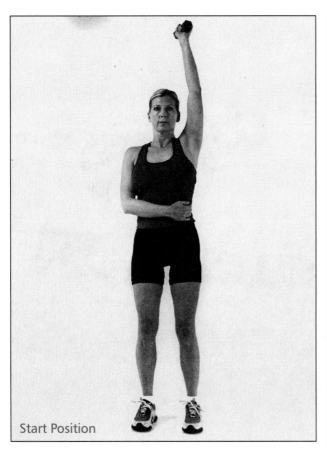

Start Position

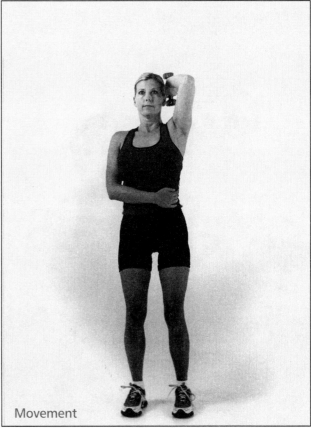

Movement

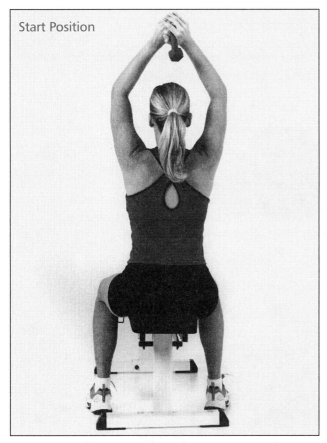

Start Position

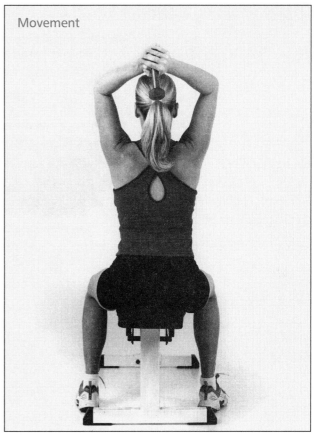

Movement

Seated Two-Arm Triceps Extensions

■ ■ ■ This exercise affects the entire triceps area. Be extra careful not to let the elbows wander away from the sides of your head during the movement.

Start Position Sit on the floor or on the edge of an exercise bench with your feet flat on the floor. Put your arms straight up, behind and over your head while holding a light dumbbell in both hands. Your palms should be facing up with your fingers spread under the weight and your thumbs crossed.

Movement Looking straight ahead, slowly lower the weight gently toward the back of your neck. Remember to keep your upper arms stable and close to the sides of your head. Do three sets of ten repetitions, resting between each set.

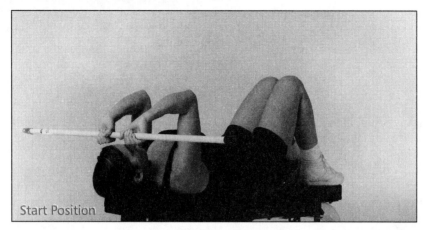

Start Position

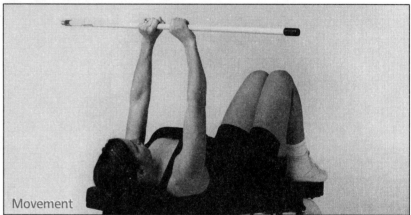

Movement

Lying Triceps Extensions

▪ ▪ ▪ This exercise is a variation of the seated extension but is performed with an unweighted straight bar.

Start Position Lie flat on an exercise bench with your knees bent and your feet up on the edge of the bench. Hold an unweighted barbell, with your hands shoulder-distance apart. Bend your elbows and hold the bar directly over your forehead.

Movement Slowly extend your arms straight up (without locking your elbows at the full extension) until the bar is directly over your eyes. Pause and slowly return the bar to the starting position. Do three sets of ten repetitions. If you are experiencing any elbow pain or discomfort, stop the exercise and consult your trainer or physician.

Close-Grip Barbell Presses

This exercise is another example of how varying your grip can place emphasis on a different muscle or part of a muscle. The classic bench press, usually for the chest, is adapted to work the triceps by using a close grip. The chest muscles will receive secondary benefit.

Start Position

Lying on a flat bench with your knees bent and your feet on the bench, grasp an unweighted bar, with your hands approximately 2 to 4 inches apart. Hold the bar just above the nipple line.

Movement

Slowly extend your arms straight up, doing the move of a classic bench press, but keeping the close grip. (The close grip puts the emphasis on the triceps muscles but gives the chest muscles benefit as well.) Pause and slowly lower the bar to the original start position. Do three sets of ten repetitions.

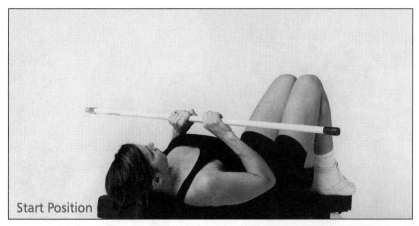

Start Position

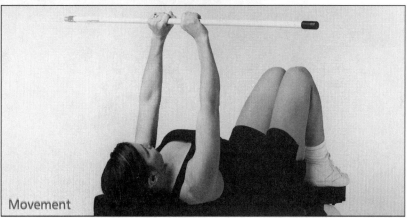

Movement

Isometric Extensions

This exercise uses isometrics, an exercise method without weights that uses muscle isolation and voluntary muscle contraction to work the muscle.

Start Position
Sit on the end of a bench or in a chair with your back straight and your shoulders rolled back. Make fists and press your upper arms straight against the sides of your body with your fists raised to chest height. Make tight fists and squeeze your triceps muscles. The effectiveness of this exercise depends on your ability to isolate the triceps muscles, visualize them working, and imagine the weight/resistance in your hands.

Movement
While concentrating on contracting the muscles, extend your lower arms straight down, pretending you are pushing down dumbbells that are in your hands. Visualize the weight in your hands and the stress on your triceps muscles. Slowly raise the arms to the start position. Do three sets of ten repetitions.

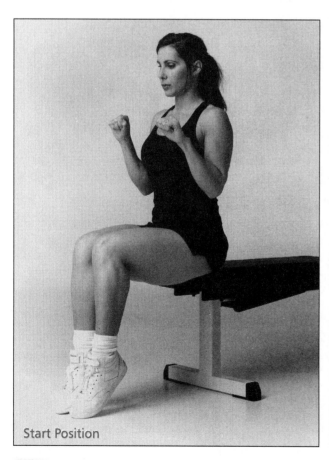
Start Position

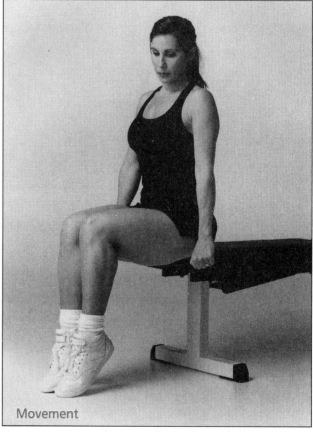
Movement

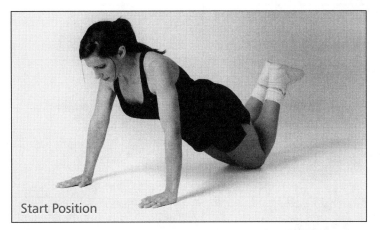

Start Position

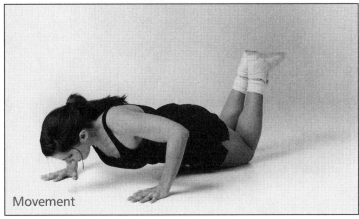

Movement

Pushups

▪ ▪ ▪ This exercise works the chest, biceps, triceps, and anterior delts—all in one exercise!

Start Position
Lie face-down on the floor with your knees on the floor and your ankles together in the air. Support your upper body with your arms perpendicular to the floor and your palms down on the floor, about shoulder-width apart. (While pushups work the entire upper body, they have particular benefit to the triceps muscles.)

Movement
Bend your arms and lower your torso until your chest touches the floor. Without resting your weight on the floor, push yourself back up to the starting position. Repeat the entire movement ten to twenty times.

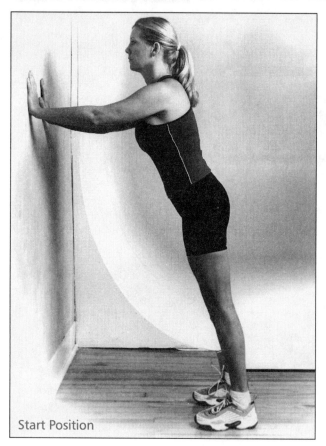

Start Position

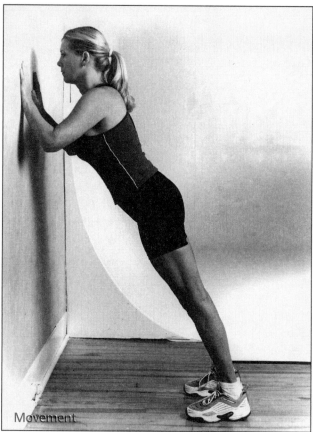

Movement

Pushups Against the Wall

■ ■ ■   This exercise is an easier version of the pushup on the floor. Beginners might find this one more user-friendly until they gain some upper-body strength.

Start Position   Stand about 3 feet away from a wall with your feet shoulder-width apart and flat on the floor. Roll your shoulders back, straighten your back, and tuck in your abs by pulling them inward toward your spine. Place your hands on the wall at shoulder height with your palms pressing on the wall.

Movement   Bend your elbows and while keeping your back straight, lean in to the wall until your upper arms are parallel to the wall. Slowly press yourself away from the wall by straightening your arms. Do three sets of ten repetitions.

Sculpting the Forearms

Have you ever heard a friend complain about his or her "out of shape forearm"? The answer is probably not, so you may wonder why we would devote any time to exercises for a body part that nobody seems to care about. The quick answer is that in any body-shaping effort, proportion is important. In other words, you would not want to put a lot of effort into building up your upper body while neglecting your entire lower body. In the same vein, if you want to develop shapely, strong arms, you cannot ignore the entire lower half.

The forearm is one of the most neglected body parts when it comes to body shaping. Because it isn't typically a trouble area, most people simply don't think about pinpointing it for exercise. As stated before, the forearm receives a minor workout in just performing most strengthening exercises for the arm, as these muscles control your grip and wrist action. However, this secondary exercise isn't enough if one of the goals of your body-shaping plan is to gain overall strength.

Think about how often you use your hands and wrists. If you work at a computer all day, you've no doubt felt the strain placed on your wrists and hands at the end of the day. What are your recreational hobbies? If you play baseball, golf, tennis, or participate in gymnastics, you are constantly relying on the strength of your wrists to carry you through the sport. And don't forget the strength of your grip! Many daily activities from picking up the kids to grocery shopping require a certain amount of strength in your grip. Several of the body-shaping exercises you will be employing also rely on your grip and wrist strength to perform them correctly. All of these things will benefit from exercising the forearms. Once you are able to recognize the need for strength in the muscles of your forearm, you will be more apt to give it the attention it deserves.

Wrist Curls

If you are a beginner, you may want to try this exercise using only one working hand at a time. The nonworking hand can be holding the working hand's forearm for support.

Start Position Sit comfortably on a flat bench while gently holding light dumbbells in your hands, palms up. Lean forward from your hips and rest your forearms on top of your thighs with your wrists hanging over the edges past your knees.

Movement Bend your wrists and bring the weights toward you within your comfortable range of motion. Make sure to relax your upper arms and keep your forearms in contact with your legs. Lower slowly. Do three sets of ten repetitions for each arm.

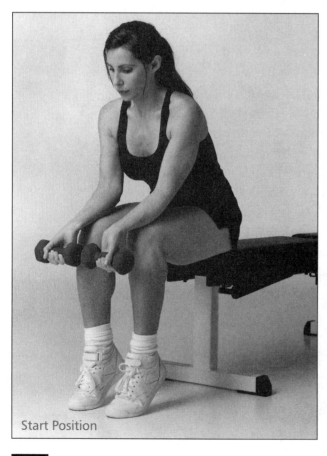

Start Position

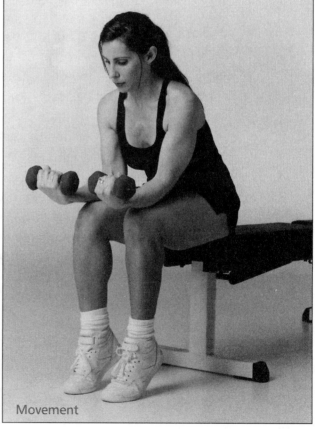

Movement

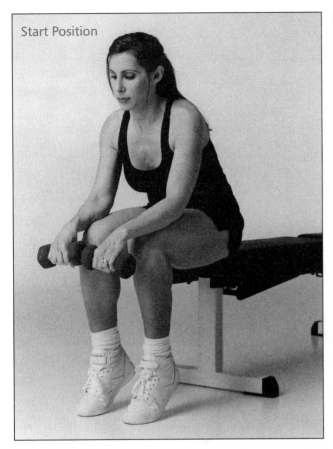

Start Position

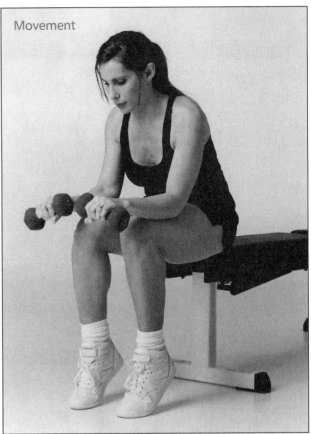

Movement

Reverse Wrist Curls

■ ■ ■ Performing this version of the previous exercise in advance ensures a full development of all sides of the forearm muscles. Again, if you are a beginner, you can perform this one hand at a time.

Start Position Sit comfortably on a flat bench while gently holding light dumbbells in your hands, palms down. Lean forward from your hips and rest your forearms on top of your thighs with your wrists hanging over the edges past your knees.

Movement Bend your wrists and bring the weights toward you within your comfortable range of motion. If your wrist bothers you, try bending it in a slightly smaller range of motion. Keep your forearms in contact with your leg. Lower your wrists slowly. Don't forget to breathe! Do two sets of ten repetitions.

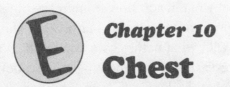

Chapter 10

Chest

If your body-shaping plan includes a goal of creating a symmetrical and balanced form, you will likely want to add chest exercises to your routine. To have a nicely toned chest simply adds to the effect of fit arms and shoulders.

Women and Chest Exercises

"We must, we must, we must increase our bust." How many of you recall this chant from your preadolescent years? It was usually sung accompanied by an isometric-type arm motion that would supposedly increase the size of your breasts. Don't get your hopes up—there is actually nothing in this book that will tell you how to increase the size of your breasts. No exercise can increase the size of your breasts. Short of implants or pills, you are stuck with what nature gave you (or didn't give you, as the case may be). However, there is something in this book that is just as valuable to you in terms of looking good, and that is a chapter devoted to exercises to build up the chest muscles under the breasts.

Breasts are basically composed of fatty tissue, which is why significant weight gain increases breast size. While exercise cannot change the size of your breasts, it can play a significant role in the appearance of your chest area. The fact is, you don't need to have large breasts to have a sexy, beautifully sculpted chest. Whether you have large or small breasts, the bottom line is that if your goal is to have a well-balanced and toned body, you will need to include the chest in your personal body-shaping program.

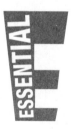

Building up the chest muscles is like having the ultimate support bra—the stronger the muscles under the breasts are, the more support they provide the fatty breast tissue, and the more the breasts are lifted for a tight and toned appearance.

Small and Large Breasts Alike

Basically, the effort you put into developing your chest muscles will result in a better-looking chest because the stronger muscles will actually hold up and lift the breasts, making them appear firmer and tighter. Women with smaller breasts will love the "line" that develops down the center of the chest, between the breasts. This "line" is not an actual line—but a slight indentation that is formed by the increase in size and definition of the muscles on either side (more detail and explanation on this later in the chest anatomy section). This line creates the illusion of cleavage for small-breasted women who normally would have no cleavage because their breasts are too small to create cleavage on their own. Likewise, larger-breasted women will develop this line and for them the line helps to create the look of firm, tight, and defined breasts.

For those of you who are overweight, some of your excess weight is being held in your breasts, so as you work out and diet, you will lose the extra fat and your breasts will start to get smaller. This isn't a bad thing! As you develop the muscles underneath, the breasts will be lifted and eventually the entire chest area will look well formed and toned.

A Word of Comfort

Don't hesitate to include the chest when you pick which body parts you want to include in your body-shaping program. If you are reluctant to work the chest because you have scary visions of the male and female bodybuilders you have seen with their rock-solid but flat breast area, don't be afraid. Be assured that this program will not do that to your body.

Those bodybuilders diet to the point of almost zero body fat so that their muscles "pop." They have an incredibly intense and rigorous workout schedule with very heavy weights and advanced training principles. Women cannot develop muscles to that degree without the use of some kind of artificial stimulus, such as steroid use.

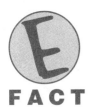

FACT

If you are a man, building the chest muscles is likely already a part of your body-shaping plan. Traditionally, a well-toned chest is a sign of strength and virility in a man. Not to mention it is also considered one of the sexiest muscle groups for a man.

Anatomy of the Chest

Your chest muscles include the pectoralis major and the pectoralis minor, known collectively as the "pecs." They are located in the upper anterior chest just under the breasts and their main function is in the movement of the upper arms.

The pectoralis major is a large "fan-shaped" muscle that is closer to the surface. Part of the pectoralis major attaches to the collarbone and runs to the upper arm in a horizontal direction. The pectoralis major works together with your shoulder muscles to move your arms forward, upward, and across the front of your body and to rotate your arms inward.

The other part of the pectoralis major runs from the sternum, or breastbone, in the center of your chest, across your chest, and up to the top of your upper arm in a diagonal direction. When you press your arms downward and inward, you contract these muscles. The pectoralis minor is underneath the pectoralis major.

Because the pectorals spread out like a fan over the rib cage, when each side is developed, they "expand" over the rib cage. There is a line down the center of the pecs, which is where the muscle is attached to the rib cage in the front. When the pecs are developed, this increases the deepness of the line, which in turn creates the illusion of deep cleavage for women.

Exercises for the Chest

If done regularly, the following exercises will provide you with a toned and well-formed chest, further improving upon the overall shape of your body. Try to visualize what you want your chest to look like. Keep this image in mind as you work out.

Do's and Don'ts

Before beginning the exercises, take a few moments to review some general exercise do's and don'ts:

- **Warm up.** Do light aerobics and stretch before working out to prepare your body for the exercises to come.
- **Follow a routine.** Set aside a quiet place and a regular time for your workout.
- **Take it easy.** Don't overtrain any body part. Avoid injury by "listening" to your body.
- **Visualize.** Concentrate on the muscle being worked—"see it" contract and tighten in your mind's eye.
- **Breathe.** Continue with regular breathing as you work out. Avoid the tendency to hold your breath as you exert yourself.

Dumbbell Presses on a Bench or Mat

This exercise is body-shaping's version of the classic "bench press."

Start Position

Holding the dumbbells in your hands, lie down flat on the floor with your knees bent, abs tucked in, and your feet on the floor or bench. Be careful getting into position while holding the weights. You may want to put yourself in a seated position first, then pick up the weights and lie down on the floor. Once in position, bend your elbows, and hold the weights with your palms facing your feet.

Movement

Slowly raise the weights straight up and slightly inward to a point straight above the center of your chest, right over your chest line. Concentrate on squeezing your chest muscles together as you raise your arms and then pause at the top for three seconds. Slowly lower the dumbbells to the start position and then repeat the movement for a total of ten repetitions. Do three sets of ten repetitions.

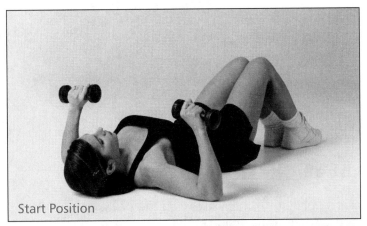

Start Position

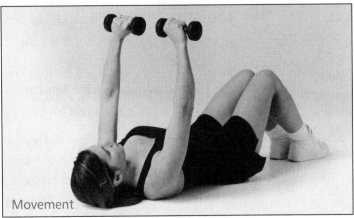

Movement

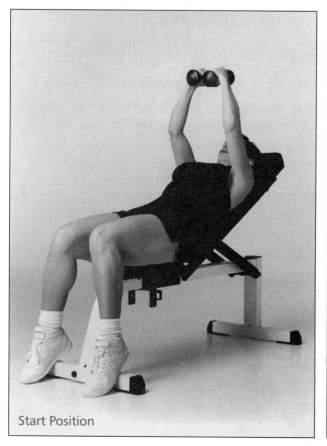

Start Position

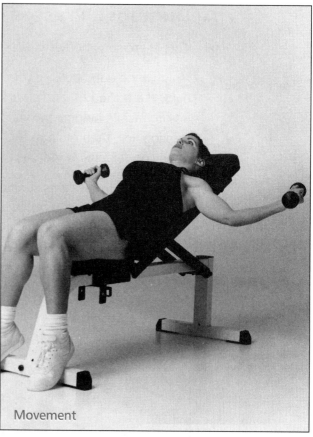

Movement

Dumbbell Chest Flyes

■ ■ ■ This exercise places primary stress on the pecs, but also has some secondary effect on the front of the deltoid (shoulder) muscle. If you want to increase the effect of this exercise and are fortunate enough to have an adjustable bench or access to a gym, perform it on an incline.

Start Position Holding the dumbbells in your hands, lie on your back on a mat or bench with your knees bent and your feet on the floor or bench. Extend your arms straight up with your palms slightly turned in to face each other.

Movement Slowly lower your arms out to the sides of your body (with your arms at right angles to your torso) as far as possible. Your elbows should remain slightly bent, or "unlocked," during the exercise. Raise your arms to the start position and repeat the movement ten times. Do three sets of ten repetitions. Start with 5-pound weights. After three or four weeks you may be ready to use 8-pounders.

Forearm Touches

This exercise is great for developing the "line" down the center of your rib cage between the two sides of the pectoral muscles. If you look at pictures of bodybuilder women in fitness magazines, this line will be apparent to you.

Start Position

Sit on a chair or bench and roll back your shoulders and tuck in your tummy. Bend your elbows with a 5-pound dumbbell in each hand, your palms facing forward, and your upper arms perpendicular to the sides of your body.

Movement

Slowly bring your forearms together to meet in front of your chest in the middle of your breasts. At the top of the movement, your palms and the dumbbells will be facing each other. Try to touch your elbows together. Hold the position for three seconds and concentrate on feeling the muscles in the middle of your chest and in the shoulders—try to feel them contract and tighten. Slowly return to the start position and repeat ten times. Do three sets of ten repetitions.

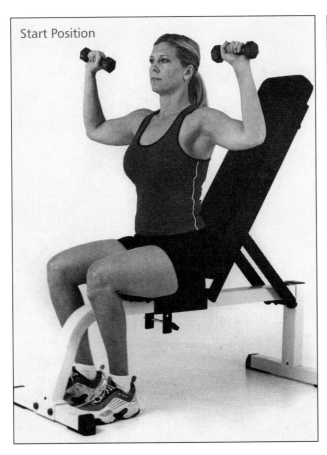

Start Position

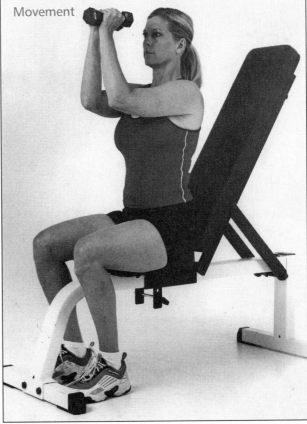

Movement

Chapter 11

Back

This chapter covers a body part that is usually neglected or at most given very little attention. When you look in the mirror, you don't see your back, so it's easy to overlook the need to shape this area. However, just because you don't see it doesn't mean you shouldn't work it! Remember that other people see it all the time!

Reasons for Sculpting the Back

A well-conditioned back not only looks great but is important for health reasons, too. Weak back muscles will cause fatigue because they cannot support the spine all day. Lower-back pain can be alleviated to a great extent by strengthening the muscles that support the lower back. Studies have shown that back-strengthening exercises provide protection against the risk of spinal fractures in those at risk for osteoporosis.

Strengthening your back muscles will also improve your posture. As you build the muscles in your back, these muscles will pull your shoulders back, thus straightening your spine. As an added bonus, when the muscles pull your shoulders back, your chest responds by protruding slightly, thus showing off that well-defined chest you've worked so hard for.

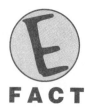

FACT

Strengthening your back muscles will also improve your posture and thereby improve your overall appearance dramatically. Better posture will also cut down on the amount of tension that is placed on your back, thus reducing the amount of lower-back pain.

Everyday Function

If you have ever had a bad back or even sore back muscles, you know how much stress is placed on the back in everyday life. The back isn't thought of very often, yet it plays an important role in everything you do. From sitting up to lifting heavy packages, the back does more than its fair share of the work. Try to pick up your crying child with a sore back, and you'll soon realize how necessary it is to keep your back in good physical condition. By adding a back-shaping routine to your exercise plan, you will increase and improve the body's function in daily activities such as lifting, carrying heavy weight, or any pulling function.

Strong and Sexy

A strong back is sexy, too. Back-baring gowns and tops are very dramatic, and strong, well-toned back muscles only increase the drama.

When you wear a bathing suit, a sculpted and toned back completes the picture that your shapely legs and arms have started. A good, strong, attractive back can be appreciated by all those you are walking away from. As a matter of fact, it is easier to be admired as you walk away because your admirer can openly gawk without fear of getting caught. A strong, sculpted back will increase the beauty of your rear view! Keep in mind that a dramatic exit can be just as impressive as a dramatic entrance.

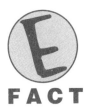

FACT

A strong and well-defined back adds to the V shape most people yearn for. Because you are building muscle, the back and shoulders will seem to be broader, thus making the waist look even smaller. A V-shaped physique is often thought of as both healthy and sexy.

Anatomy of the Back

Before you dive in to the exercises, it is always good to have an idea of exactly what muscles you will be working. The following sections will give a brief explanation of the muscles of the back. As you are working out, try to concentrate on each of these muscle groups. As you know, visualization can help tremendously when it comes to spot sculpting.

The Trapezius

The trapezius (commonly known as the "traps") muscle is a flat, triangular muscle that extends out and down from the neck and then down between the shoulder blades. It is located just beneath the skin, so if you touch around back there, you will be able to feel this muscle. Its basic function is to support the shoulders. However, the traps also aid in turning or tilting the head, shrugging the shoulders, and twisting and raising the arms. Though this muscle is often considered to be a shoulder muscle as opposed to a back muscle, it is included here since you will be working the traps as you do the exercises within this chapter.

The Latissimi Dorsi

The latissimi dorsi (commonly known as the "lats") are the large triangular muscles that extend from under the shoulders down the small of the back on both sides. These are the largest muscles of the upper body. They function to pull the shoulders down and to the back. You use the lats when you go swimming or reach up and pull something down that is higher than your head.

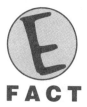

FACT

The latissimi dorsi are now being used to form new breasts in those who have suffered breast cancer. Basically, the muscle is cut away and brought around underneath the armpit to the front of the body where it is positioned to create a new breast.

The Spinal Erectors

The spinal erectors are several muscles in the lower back that guard the nerve channels and help keep the spine erect. As its name suggests, the main job of the spinal erectors is to hold the spine erect. Because the spinal erectors support the upper body, it is very important that you do not overdo any exercises for the back. As you can imagine, almost all exercises are going to require the use of the spinal erectors, so they get a pretty good workout even when they aren't targeted. They are the slowest muscles in the body to recover from heavy exercise.

Exercises for the Back

Whether you are looking to shape the ideal body or simply want a healthier body, working the back muscles is always a good idea. The back muscles play an important role in our everyday lives. There simply isn't much we can do if our back is out of commission. Therefore, it is very important that you read the exercise descriptions carefully and peruse the pictures provided to make sure that you are doing the exercise correctly and in the proper form. The last thing you want to do is injure your back. Abdominal strength is also important. The abs oppose the back muscles and if one is weaker or stronger than the other, the resulting muscle imbalance can potentially aid in injury.

Do's and Don'ts

Before beginning the exercises, take a few moments to review some general exercise do's and don'ts:

- **Warm up.** Do light aerobics and stretch before working out to prepare your body for the exercises to come.
- **Follow a routine.** Set aside a quiet place and a regular time for your workout.
- **Take it easy.** Don't overtrain any body part. Avoid injury by "listening" to your body.
- **Visualize.** Concentrate on the muscle being worked—"see it" contract and tighten in your mind's eye.
- **Breathe.** Continue with regular breathing as you work out. Avoid the tendency to hold your breath as you exert yourself.

Your back is constantly working. Whether you are walking, running, or simply standing up straight, your back is supporting the movement and balance of your body. Add to that all the little chores we complete every day, such as picking up the baby or pulling the car door shut, and you can easily see why back strength is needed and how back pain is often caused. Many people suffer from back pain, whether constant or just every once in a while. The best way to combat this is to exercise the back on a regular basis. As you add strength and build muscle, your back is better able to handle everyday chores without strain or probability of injury. That said, if you do suffer back pain of any sort, be sure to check with your health care provider before participating in any exercise regimen. He or she will be able to advise you on those exercises you should and should not do in regards to your particular back condition.

Bent-Over Rowing with Unweighted Bar

This exercise strengthens the upper back and erector spinal. Along with developed shoulders, this back exercise will help you achieve that "V" look to your upper body.

Start Position Stand with your feet shoulder-width apart, holding an unweighted bar. Unlock your knees and bend forward slightly until your back is almost parallel to the floor. Extend your arms downward with your palms facing to the back. Keep your abs tucked in throughout the entire exercise.

Movement Concentrate on the middle traps between your shoulder blades so you can feel them contract as you slowly pull the unweighted bar straight up until it lightly touches your chest. "Pinch" your shoulder blades together and hold the position for three seconds. Then slowly lower the bar to the original position. Repeat for three sets of ten repetitions.

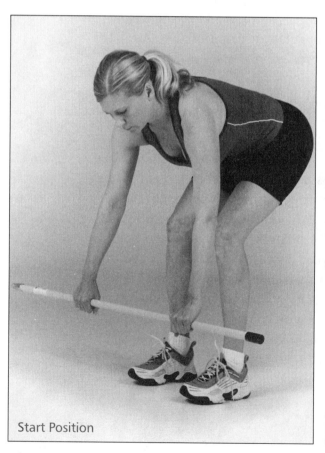

Start Position

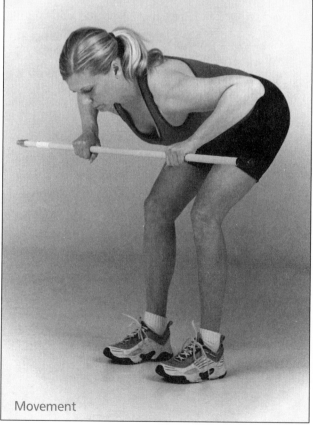

Movement

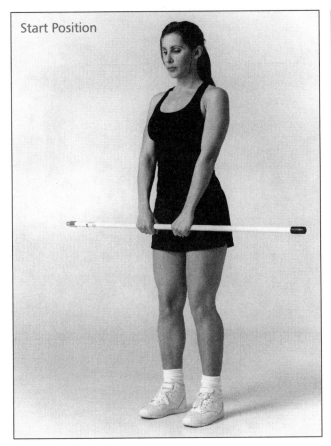

Start Position

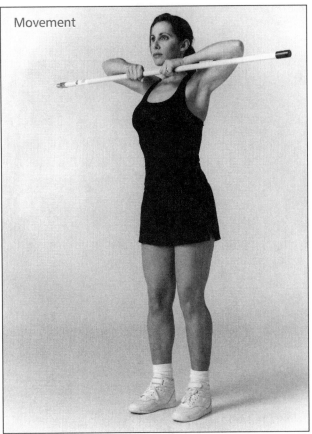

Movement

Upright Rowing

The purpose of this exercise is to develop the trap, but it has a great effect on the front lateral deltoids as well. It also helps create definition in your shoulders, or striation, between the deltoids and the pecs.

Start Position Stand with your feet slightly apart and your arms down in front of you, holding a light unweighted bar. Place your hands about 12 inches apart, palms facing your body. Unlock your knees, tuck in your abs, and roll your shoulders back.

Movement Slowly pull the bar up until it almost touches your chin. As you pull up, keep your elbows up above your ears and your shoulders down. When the bar is at the top of the movement, hold the position for three seconds and feel your trapezius muscles contract; then slowly lower the bar to the start position. Perform this movement for a total of three sets of ten repetitions each.

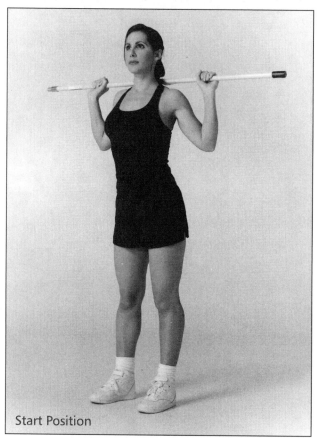

Start Position

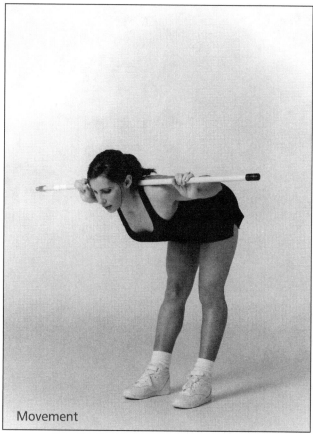

Movement

Good Mornings

So called because the movement resembles a person bowing "good morning," this exercise isolates the lower back muscles.

Start Position Stand with your feet slightly apart. Hold an unweighted bar across the back of your shoulders.

Movement Keeping your legs and back straight, bend forward from the waist, head up, until your torso is almost parallel to the floor. Hold for three seconds, then slowly come back up to the start position. Repeat ten times for three sets of ten repetitions.

Deadlifts

· · · Deadlifts are an overall power exercise that work much more than just your lower back, which receives the primary benefit. Your trapezius muscles, buttocks, and even your leg muscles are working in this movement.

Start Position Stand with your feet shoulder-width apart. Place an unweighted bar on the floor in front of you. Roll your shoulders back and tuck in your stomach. Bend at the knees, lean forward, and grasp the bar with a medium-wide, overhand grip.

Movement Keep your eyes focused straight ahead. Do not look down when performing this movement. By driving with your legs, straighten up until you are standing upright. With the bar resting lightly against your thighs, roll your shoulders back and throw your chest out; hold that position for a few seconds before slowly lowering the bar to the floor by bending your knees and leaning forward from the waist. Do two sets of ten repetitions.

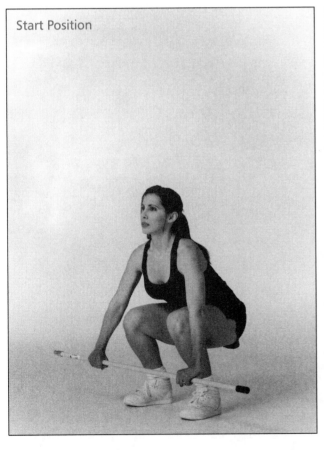
Start Position

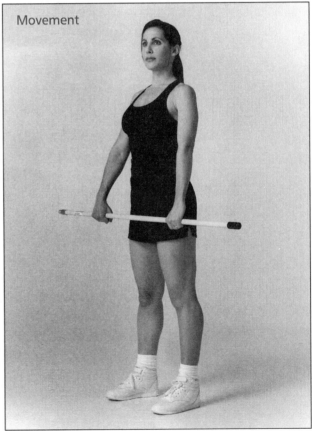
Movement

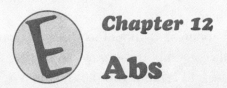

Chapter 12

Abs

Of all the body parts, the abdominal muscles are those that need targeting exercises the most, because the abdomen contains muscles that don't "work" otherwise. While our arms and legs get at least some kind of workout during daily activity, the stomach muscles will steadily grow weaker if not specifically worked. This chapter will show you how to sculpt those troublesome abs.

Dieting While Working the Abs

A belly bulge can plague even those who are not overweight and have never felt the need to diet. Think of how many times you have noticed a slim woman only to be surprised to see a protruding belly when she wears a tight outfit. Women who have borne children also have a great need to strengthen their poor overworked and stretched-out abdominal muscles. Body fat has a way of settling in the abdomen.

In earlier chapters, much has been said about the ability of body-shaping techniques to do what diets cannot do—change the shape of the body. However, this is a good place to remind you that it is important to realize that in the world of body shaping, the stomach is one body part for which improvement requires an equal effort in dieting.

Dieting as an Adjunct

Elsewhere in this book we have talked about dieting as an adjunct, to help show off the body shaping you have done. The point has been made that it is possible to reshape areas such as the arms and legs by targeting them with specific exercises and that this will accomplish what all the diets in the world will not do. However, we have to vary that stand a bit when it comes to the abdominals. You can do abdominal exercises for an hour a day, every day, for months, and you will never see the muscles that have developed under the layer of fat on your belly! This isn't to say your work won't get you results—you just won't be able to see them. Working the abs will build and tone the muscles, but no amount of exercise will magically remove the fat that covers the muscles in this area. You will have to work to reduce overall body fat, and particularly in the belly area, in order to reveal the toned muscles in your abs.

Dieting Alone Doesn't Work

On the flip side, let's remember why diet alone does not work. Restricting caloric consumption (or fat, or carbs—whatever diet you prefer) may get rid of the layer of fat, but the abdominals that are then revealed will not be developed, toned, or well shaped. Therefore, if you do still have some body fat to lose, don't wait until you lose it to start working the abs. Even though you may not see the results right away, begin your ab program with determination so that when you do lose the desired amount of fat, you will see the results of the work you have been doing all along.

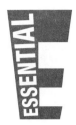

Most of the exercises for the other body parts in this book contain a reminder to "tuck in your stomach" or "pull in your abs." To do this, imagine you are wearing an old-fashioned corset and you are pulling your stomach in to lace up the strings. By doing this, you will be accomplishing double duty—giving your ab muscles a work out, too!

Successful Abdominal Routines

Exercises for the abs are usually best done without using weights. If you train the abs with weight, they might get thicker and bigger. This is one case where increasing the size of the muscle is a disadvantage, because thicker and larger ab muscles might actually give the appearance of a protruding belly. High repetition is the secret to a successful abdominal routine.

Exercise experts differ on the subject of how often you should work the abs. Many maintain that you should rest muscle groups and work them only every other day, and you should treat the abs like every other muscle group in this respect. Others, however, believe that daily exercise of the abs is the way to go and that the need to rest your muscles is just a myth. Even some bodybuilders, who do adhere to the alternating workout style, exempt the abs from the resting pattern and work them every day.

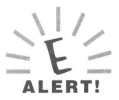

It is very easy to forget to breathe while doing abdominal exercises. As you already know, it is essential that you breathe. If you are having difficulty remembering to breathe, count your reps out loud. This will force you to inhale and exhale appropriately.

Because the abdominal muscles are "core" muscles—meaning they are located in the torso and are holding you upright (along with the back muscles)—they are constantly working. It is true that resistance training with weights should be done on alternate days to allow for muscle recovery. The exception with the abs is due to the fact that they are not trained with weights and are essential to overall postural health and well-being. If muscle soreness is felt for more than two days, too much has been done.

Anatomy of the Abdominal Muscles

There are four major muscles that form what is known as the "abs," or the abdominal muscle group: the rectus abdominus, external oblique, internal oblique, and transversus abdominus.

The rectus abdominus is a long vertical muscle that runs the length of your torso, originating just above the pubic bone and ending in the lower ribs. It is a long, wide, flat sheet of muscle commonly referred to in parts: the lower and upper abs. This muscle is used to provide stability to your torso when you bend forward. Many people mistake this muscle as being two. While you can certainly use differing movements to accentuate either the upper or lower sections, it is actually all one big muscle; therefore, any movement you do will affect the whole thing.

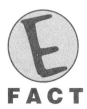

FACT

Core training refers to working on the group of muscles that make up the center of the body—the abs and the back. There are "core" classes specifically geared to strengthening this area of the body to improve sports performance, back and spinal health, balance, and posture.

On either side of this long muscle are the obliques. The external oblique muscle is a broad, thin muscle that runs in a diagonal line from your ribs to your hip. The internal oblique muscle is under the external and runs at right angles to it. In fact, the degree of slant at which these two muscles meet is what determines the size and shape of your waist. These are the muscles you use when you twist or bend to the side. Developing these muscles helps to give your waist that desirable tapered look.

The transversus abdominus is the deepest-set ab muscle and runs horizontally underneath the rectus abdominus. This muscle is the one you feel when you exhale forcefully, cough, or sneeze. This muscle acts as a stabilizer and thus receives a workout along with pretty much any other ab exercises you do.

Exercises for the Abs

This is one of the most commonly worked muscle groups simply because toned abs are sexy and can create a great overall appearance. Whether you want to show off your efforts or simply feel better about yourself, working the abs is a great addition to your body-shaping plan.

Fitness experts debate the proper position of the hands while doing crunches. Some say to keep your hands on your chest when doing any type of crunch, not behind your head in classic sit-up style. They argue that when your hands are behind your head, you may pull your neck forward to assist in the crunch movement, not only threatening to injure your neck muscles, but also diminishing the amount of work your ab muscles are doing. However, others argue that the hands should be placed behind the head while doing crunches to give the neck support. Use whichever position you are most comfortable with.

Do's and Don'ts

Before beginning the exercises, take a few moments to review some general exercise do's and don'ts:

- **Warm up.** Do light aerobics and stretch before working out to prepare your body for the exercises to come.
- **Follow a routine.** Set aside a quiet place and a regular time for your workout.
- **Take it easy.** Don't overtrain any body part. Avoid injury by "listening" to your body.
- **Visualize.** Concentrate on the muscle being worked—"see it" contract and tighten in your mind's eye.
- **Breathe.** Continue with regular breathing as you work out. Avoid the tendency to hold your breath as you exert yourself.

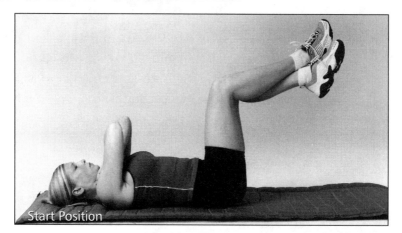

Start Position

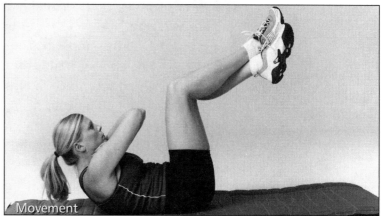

Movement

Classic Crunches

This exercise works the upper and lower abs, the rectus abdominus.

Start Position   Lie on your back on a mat on the floor. Raise your legs with your knees bent and cross your ankles. Cross your hands over your chest. Keep the small of your back pressed firmly against the floor during this exercise.

Movement   Raise your upper body toward your knees while simultaneously bringing your knees in toward your chest. Try to get your shoulder blades off the floor. Feel the contraction in the abdominals as the upper and lower body "crunch" together. At the top of the movement, hold the position for three seconds and give your abs an extra "crunch," for maximum effect. Make sure you do not hold your breath! Repeat for a total of two or three sets of ten repetitions each.

Oblique Crunches

This variation of the classic crunch exercise works both the obliques and the lower abs.

Start Position

Lie on your back on a mat on the floor with your knees bent and your feet flat on the floor. Cross your arms over your chest with your palms flat against your shoulders. Lift your right foot and lay it on top of your left knee.

Movement

Perform the "crunch" movement, curling your shoulders upward and rotating your torso to the side toward your right raised knee. Repeat for a total of ten repetitions, then switch to the other side by placing your left foot on your right knee, and do another ten repetitions. Do two sets of ten repetitions.

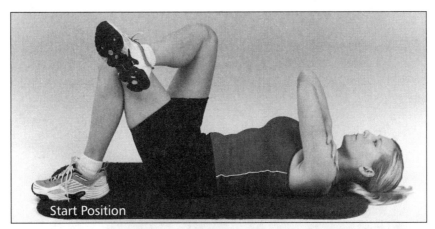

Start Position

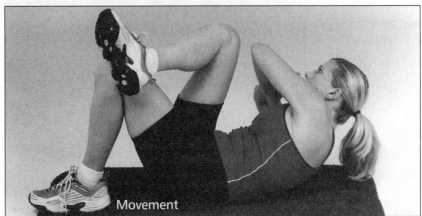

Movement

Knee-Up Leg Raises

■ ■ ■   This exercise targets the lower abs.

Start Position Lie flat on your back on a mat on the floor. Your arms should be at your sides with your hands placed palms down under your buttocks (this helps keep the small of your lower back pressed against the floor during the movement). Keep your upper body and feet a few inches off the floor during the entire exercise to maintain tension in the abs.

Movement Slowly bend your knees, pulling them up toward your chest. Hold that position for three seconds and feel the muscles in your abs contract. Lower your legs to the start position. Do two sets of twelve repetitions.

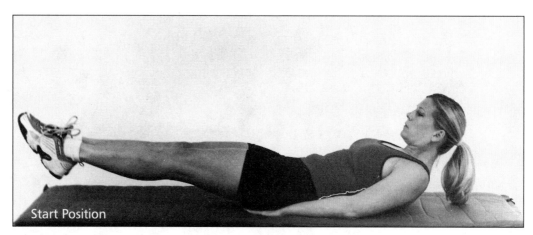

Start Position

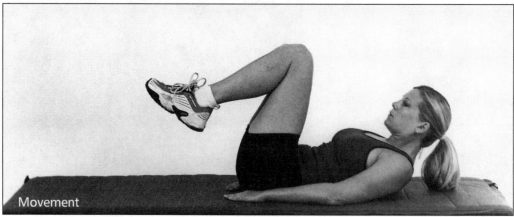

Movement

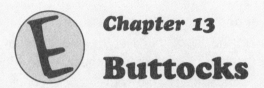

Chapter 13

Buttocks

Although diet and exercise can help you lose weight and lessen the overall size of your buttocks, the only way to see a real difference in the shape of the lower body is to body shape. This chapter will show you how to use targeted resistance exercises to get the shapely buttocks you've dreamed of.

Reasons for Sculpting the Buttocks

Nearly everyone can come up with a good reason to sculpt the buttocks. Even those people who seem to have the perfect backside often have to work hard to achieve that look. While you may not give your backside a lot of attention, just think about all the attention it gets from others. Purposely or not, other people look at your backside as you walk away from them, leave a room, or turn a corner. Also, considering that the buttocks are viewed as one of the "sexy" parts of the body in today's society, you are likely to get a good once-over from those attracted to you. Perhaps you aren't as vain as most of us, and your buttocks concern stems from the simple fact that your clothes don't fit comfortably. Whatever your reason for wanting to sculpt the buttocks, this chapter can help you out.

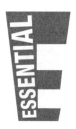

Because genetics partially determine the size of your buttocks, you need to maintain reasonable body-shaping goals. If you have wide hips and a curvy body, you will simply have to shape a posterior that fits in well with your body's proportions. You cannot change genetics, but you can tone and tighten your way to a beautiful and healthy physique.

Pinpointing the Problem

Take a look in the mirror, this time focusing on your backside. Since this is an area that isn't easily seen by you, it is easy to neglect it. Take a long hard look. Try to get the best view possible. If you aren't able to get a good full view of your backside, you may want to ask a trusted friend to give you a good once-over. However, be sure this friend feels comfortable being open and honest with you. Brutal honesty is what you're looking for here. You have to be able to identify the problem before you can work to rectify it.

Now, take note of what you (or your friend) saw. Did your butt look too saggy? Did it seem too big and out of proportion with the rest of your body? Perhaps you don't have much of a tush to speak of. Whatever the problem, body shaping can help solve it.

The Body-Shaping Solution

For those of you suffering a saggy backside, it's likely that age and gravity have taken their tolls on you. But don't fret; what was once saggy can yet be perky again! As you get older, a lot of parts of your body will start to droop—the breasts, facial skin, eyelids, and, of course, the buttocks. This is just a part of nature. However, plastic surgery aside, you can do your part through exercise to help avoid or counteract the effect of aging on your backside. By toning, building, and strengthening the muscles in your butt, you can give that saggy posterior a natural lift.

If you looked and looked and still could not find your butt, don't worry; you aren't alone. A lot of people have the flat butt look. While a flat butt may seem like a blessing to those of you looking to shed a few pounds off the posterior, those who have a flat butt know that it can be a curse. A flat butt can create a look of ill proportion, especially if the front side of the body is voluptuous, and clothes may not fit very well (fitted in other areas and saggy in the buttock region). The best way to beat a flat butt is to body shape. By toning and building the muscles in the buttocks, you can give your butt more shape and a rounded appearance.

Some of you may just think your butt is too big overall. This is a common complaint, as the body tends to store fat in the buttock area. This natural fat reserve provides a cushion for the pelvic bone, so it does actually have a function; it's not just there to annoy you. If this is your posterior view, then you will likely need to add an aerobic segment to your body-shaping plan. Again, aerobic exercise and a sensible diet will help you to lose that layer of fat that is covering the muscles you are working. While you cannot target specific areas of fat, you can target specific muscles. Therefore, while you are using aerobics and diet to reduce the amount of fat in the buttocks, continue to work the buttock muscles as well. The end result will be a shapely, perky, and well-toned butt that you will take pride in and want to show off.

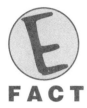

FACT

When you work your glutes, you not only accomplish a change in the shape of the area; you also affect other health factors. Strong glutes support your back better, increase your leg endurance in sports, and help reduce lower-back pain.

Anatomy of the Buttocks

The gluteus muscles of the buttock area, or "glutes" as they are commonly called, form the largest muscle group in the body (that's not a very comforting thought!) and are located at the base of the back. The gluteus maximus, the medius, and the minimus are the three parts of this muscle group. The maximus (largest, as the name implies) is used when you walk, run, and jump. The gluteus maximus runs from the hipbone to the tailbone, and works to extend and rotate the thigh. The medius assists in more lateral movements used in such activities as skating, tennis, or basketball. The minimus is the smallest of the three. When you rotate your leg outward from the hip, you use your gluteus minimus. This is the muscle that is underneath the notorious "saddlebag" that some people have.

Cardio Programs Benefit the Buttocks

While cardio programs benefit the entire body, if your buttocks and abs are trouble areas for you, you may want to seriously consider adding a cardio program to your body-shaping plan. As you learned from Chapter 12, the only way to truly get rid of that layer of fat covering your body is to burn it off. In order to do this, you must use an exercise program that increases your heart rate and gets that blood pumping. There are several methods you can choose from that will not only add an aerobic exercise, but will also give you the benefit of strengthening the buttocks.

Walking

Walking is the easiest and most popular form of exercise. Everywhere you look, people of all ages are out there walking their butts off—pun intended. This is a great form of exercise to get you out of the house and into the fresh air. Several people benefit from having walking partners. You can catch up on the latest gossip and do your body some good at the same time. However, keep in mind that you need to keep up a good pace in order to accomplish anything significant. You should be able to talk some while walking, but certainly not sing. You want to get your heart rate up enough to make you perspire and increase your body temperature.

Walking in itself helps to strengthen the buttocks, but if you really want to target them, the best way is to walk a course that has hills. After walking up hills briskly, you will certainly feel the muscles in the buttocks that have been worked. Along with strengthening the glutes, you are also working to burn off some of that extra fat!

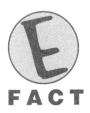

FACT

A lot of people are incorporating a power-walking routine into their exercise regimens. This is a form of walking that is done at a rapid pace. It also utilizes the arms to add even more strengthening qualities. Visit your local mall before all the shops open and you'll likely see several people power walking their way to fitness.

Hiking

Hiking is another great activity. While it might not be available to you every day, it is something you should definitely take advantage of given the chance. You can consider hiking as an advanced form of walking. Typically, a hike takes place in the woods, often on mountainsides. Because the terrain is full of obstacles, the body uses a lot of muscle to maneuver and maintain balance. If the hike is going uphill, this will really get your buttocks into shape. Also considering that hikes usually require a backpack or some other kind of additional burden, you are making your body work that much harder by adding weight. If you are the outdoorsy type, this is a good aerobic activity to take advantage of as much as possible. Not only do you get to enjoy the natural wonders of the world, but a lot of energy is required as well, giving your body a great workout.

Running/Jogging

If you'd like to pick up the pace a bit, running or jogging may be for you. This is an activity that requires no equipment but provides a great workout. (Of course, you can always use a treadmill if you prefer.) This is a little more (or a lot more, depending on how fast and far you wish to go) than walking. By picking up the pace you are making your heart and respiratory system work harder, giving you a better aerobic workout. Running and jogging also work to strengthen the glutes, especially if you add a few hills to your course. If you are particularly concerned with working the glutes, running sprints makes for an even better exercise.

Bicycling

Bike riding is an enjoyable pastime for kids and adults alike. So why not make it a part of your body-shaping plan? That's right, pull that bike out of the garage, dust it off, and go for a ride. Remember, once you've learned how to ride a bike, you never forget. Of course, you'll want to wear a helmet, just in case. If you have children, this is a great way to save time. You can take the kids out for a ride, thus spending quality time with them and getting a workout at the same time.

Riding a bike is great exercise, not only for your heart and respiratory system, but also for your thighs, hips, and most importantly, your buttocks. If you are more of an indoor person, then you can always get on the stationary bikes at the local gym. This is just as good as taking a ride around the neighborhood. You might also like to try the spinning classes offered at most local gyms.

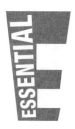

Most of us want some type of aerobic activity to burn off the layer of fat that is covering the muscles we are trying to develop. Participating in one of these activities on a regular basis will allow you to do just that and give you the added bonus of strengthening and shaping the buttocks!

Exercises for the Buttocks

Now that you have set your buttock-shaping goals, it's time to put your plan into action. The following exercises will give you a great start to toning and tightening the muscles of the buttocks. To make the most of your buttock exercises, you must focus on the muscles being worked. Concentrate on the glutes with every movement. Feel them work. You can even add a little extra quality to your workout by squeezing the muscles as you work them. It's up to you to add aerobic exercises and a sensible diet if you want to achieve the greatest results. As always, visualize what you want and then go for it!

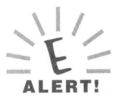

Many exercises for the buttocks require you to lift or extend your leg. Be careful not to overextend the leg during any of these exercises. Doing so will take the concentration away from the buttocks and place it on the lower back, not only rendering the exercise ineffective, but also risking injury.

Do's and Don'ts

Before beginning the exercises, take a few moments to review some general exercise do's and don'ts:

- **Warm up.** Do light aerobics and stretch before working out to prepare your body for the exercises to come.
- **Follow a routine.** Set aside a quiet place and a regular time for your workout.
- **Take it easy.** Don't overtrain any body part. Avoid injury by "listening" to your body.
- **Visualize.** Concentrate on the muscle being worked—"see it" contract and tighten in your mind's eye.
- **Breathe.** Continue with regular breathing as you work out. Avoid the tendency to hold your breath as you exert yourself.

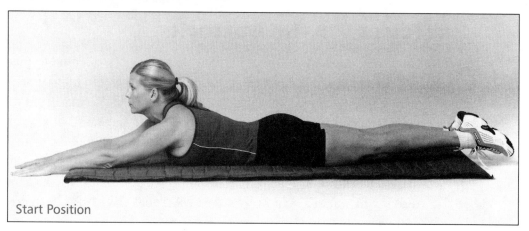

Start Position

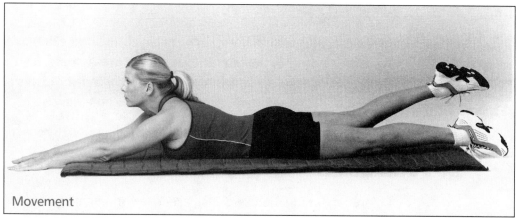

Movement

Rear Leg Scissors

This is an excellent exercise to target the buttocks and lower back.

Start Position
Lie on your stomach on a mat on the floor. Extend your arms out in front of your body and place your palms flat on the floor.

Movement
Raise your legs off the floor as much as possible. Move your feet apart a short distance, then bring them together and cross one over the other. Move them apart and cross them again with the opposite leg on top this time. Repeat this scissors motion for the required number of repetitions. Concentrate on feeling the contraction in the buttock area. Repeat ten times for each position; do three sets.

Fire Hydrants

. . . This classic does double duty—it works your hips and butt in one exercise!

Start Position   Place your body in an all-fours position, resting on your knees, arms fully extended, palms on the floor, and elbows locked. Keep your back parallel to the floor and be careful not to arch or sway it downward.

Movement   Keeping your knees bent, lift your left knee and extend it outward to the side of your body. Next, unbend your knee so your leg is extended straight out. Your leg will be extended out to your side at a 90-degree angle. Hold for three seconds and feel the muscles in your buttock contract. (You will also feel this in your outer thigh/hip area.) Return the knee to the bent position and then back to the start position. Repeat for a total of ten repetitions. Switch to the other leg and do another ten repetitions, building up to three sets for each leg.

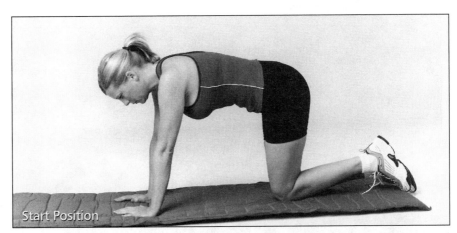

Start Position

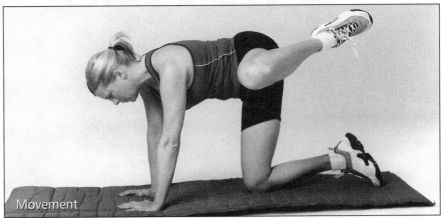

Movement

Back Leg Kicks

Use your concentration skills and really focus on the butt muscles for optimal effect.

Start Position

Place your body in the all-fours position (down on hands and knees).

Movement

Extend your right leg straight out behind you, allowing your foot to lightly touch the floor. Keep your back parallel to the floor. Lift the extended leg just above the horizontal position or to the point just before your lower back begins to arch, concentrating on the tightening feeling in the buttock area. Hold for three seconds in that position then return to the start position, but without allowing your foot to touch the floor. Without resting, repeat the movement for the required number of repetitions without letting your foot touch the floor. Do three sets of ten repetitions for each leg.

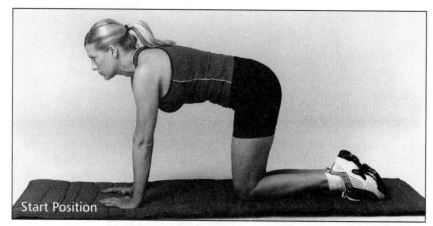

Start Position

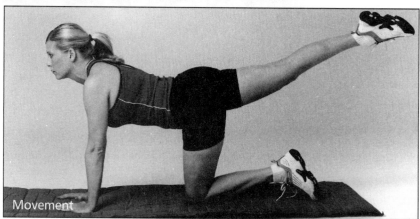

Movement

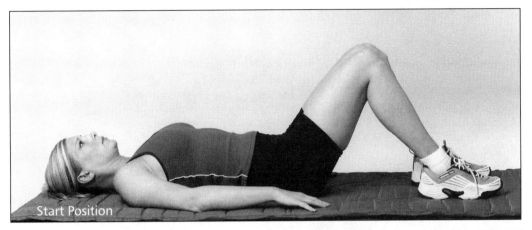

Start Position

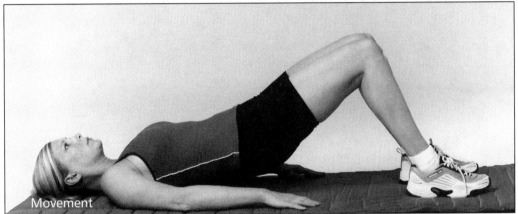

Movement

Buttock Tighteners

■ ■ ■   Holding the raised position for a few seconds—and squeezing the muscles—greatly increases the effectiveness of this movement.

Start Position   Lie on your back on a mat on the floor. Put the soles of your feet flat on the floor with your knees bent and your feet placed together and pulled up toward your butt. Place your hands out to the sides of your waist with your palms lightly resting on the floor.

Movement   Raise your butt off the floor so that your back, butt, and thighs form an almost straight line. Hold the raised position for three seconds while concentrating on tightening your butt muscles. Slowly lower yourself to the start position. Repeat for a total of three sets of ten repetitions.

Variation: Perform the same movement with your feet shoulder-width apart instead of together.

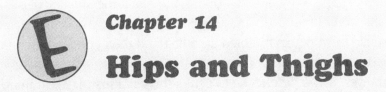

Chapter 14

Hips and Thighs

If you are tired of having a wide lower body or weak hips, then this chapter is for you. Here you will learn exercises to strengthen (and narrow) this common problem area. While aerobic activity will help shrink this area, noticeable changes in the hips and thighs can only be effected by serious resistance training, which will actually trim inches off the size.

Sculpting the Hips and Thighs

The hips and thighs tend to be a problem area for most women. (Men tend not to be bothered too much with this region.) You may be one of the many out there to flip to this section first. For some of us, it just seems as though nothing can be done until the hips and thighs are first sculpted to the ideal shape. Why bother working the abs if the smaller waist size of your jeans won't fit up over your thighs? For some of you it may just make better sense to work this troubled area first and then concentrate on the other parts of your body. Of course, the ultimate body-shaping plan is up to you. However, if you do choose to sculpt this area first, keep in mind that you aren't finished once you reach your goal. You will need to continue to work these muscles if you want to maintain the shape you created. In other words, don't expect a quick-fix miracle solution.

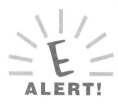

No matter how much you exercise and diet, you will never be able to change the shape of your bone structure. Therefore, if your hip bones are wide-set, then you are going to have wide hips and there's nothing you can do about it. However, by toning and strengthening the muscles of the hips, you can give the illusion of narrower hips.

Defining Your Goals

Before jumping right in to the exercises, it's a good idea to set some goals. Take a close look at your hips and thighs. What parts need to be worked? Perhaps your hips are excellent, but your thighs balloon out. In this case you would need to focus on working your upper thighs. Maybe the outside thigh muscles are toned and strong, but the inside muscles do little more than take up space. In this case you would want to concentrate on those exercises that target the inner thighs. Whatever your situation may be, you need to be aware of what exactly it is you want to accomplish before you can set forth a plan to reach your goals.

Those of you who have a "pear-shaped " figure know that weight loss alone cannot fix this problem area. Even women who do not really have that pear-shaped structure admit that the weight seems to settle in the hips and thighs before anywhere else. With a combination of aerobic exercise, a sensible diet, and targeted resistance exercises, you can change this pear shape into your ideal shape.

For most, your basic goal will be to reduce the circumference of the area. If you want to follow your progress in this area, make sure to measure your hips and thighs before you begin the program and then every three or four weeks. When you measure be sure to place the tape measure in the same spot each time. By doing these targeted exercises, you will get toned and tighter thighs and hips, allowing you to look nice in those new slacks.

Because the inner thighs are muscles that are not used much in daily activity, they tend to get flabby and only targeted exercise will tone the muscles in this area. The same principle applies to the outer thigh or "saddlebag area." While you may use your quads and glutes in moving around, climbing stairs, and so on, you don't move sideways very much, so this area tends to get loose and flabby without targeted work.

Adding Aerobics

An added word here about your aerobics portion as it applies to this body part: If you really want to increase the effectiveness of your aerobic workout for this body part, you will want to do some sort of step aerobics instead of just doing your standard aerobics program. Any aerobic activity that includes "stepping" will kick it up a notch and will result in better, faster, and more dramatic changes to your hips, thighs, and buttocks areas. Try aerobics classes that use walking and running up steps or an elliptical bike for a real blast to your hips and thighs. Stair climbers and step aerobics are excellent exercise programs for the butt, hips, and thighs because of the up-and-down motion.

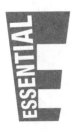

You may have heard that your butt and thighs will get bigger by working those muscles. Don't worry—it is just a myth. Unless you are using very heavy weight and low reps, you will not make the muscles larger. Instead, they will be more toned and tighter with a better shape, not larger.

Anatomy of the Hips and Thighs

Together with the muscles of the buttocks, the muscles of the hips and thighs are part of the largest muscle group of the body. The muscles that make up the hip and thigh area are called *adductors* and *abductors*.

The muscles along the inner thigh are the hip adductors. They function to move your leg across the midline of your body. The muscles in your outer thighs are called hip abductors. When you move your leg away from your body, you are using the abductors.

Strong inner and outer thigh muscles protect your knees and hips when you move from side to side. If you are a skier, tennis player, or basketball player, these muscles are particularly important to develop and strengthen to prevent injury. The inner thighs, or adductors, are like your upper arms, or triceps in the sense that both are problem "flabby" areas. Just as women don't use their triceps in natural daily activity, the same goes for the inner thighs. You don't move sideways very much, which is the movement that works the muscles of the inner thighs, so these muscles don't get much of a workout in your daily life. This is all the more reason to target this muscle for spot training. If done regularly, at least three or four times a week, you will see it tighten and it will make a difference in how your legs look.

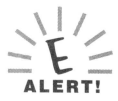

ALERT!

When doing exercises for the thighs, it is best to keep your knees unlocked. Locking the knees stresses the joints, and it also takes away the stimulation from the thigh muscles. The more you can stimulate the muscles during a workout, the greater the results you will achieve.

Exercises for the Hips and Thighs

As you know, the hips and thighs are problem areas for many women. However, keep this bright thought in mind: Women have strong legs by nature. This fact will make it easier to tone and strengthen the muscles of the legs. This isn't to say that you don't have to work hard. On the contrary, working the thigh muscles is some of the hardest work you will do in this body-shaping program. But because these muscles respond so well to exercise, you will likely end up with exactly the results you envision. So, are you ready to begin shaping those thighs and hips?

Do's and Don'ts

Before beginning the exercises, take a few moments to review some general exercise do's and don'ts:

- **Warm up.** Do light aerobics and stretch before working out to prepare your body for the exercises to come.
- **Follow a routine.** Set aside a quiet place and a regular time for your workout.
- **Take it easy.** Don't overtrain any body part. Avoid injury by "listening" to your body.
- **Visualize.** Concentrate on the muscle being worked—"see it" contract and tighten in your mind's eye.
- **Breathe.** Continue with regular breathing as you work out. Avoid the tendency to hold your breath as you exert yourself.

Because the hip and thigh area is a typical trouble zone, many people are eager to jump right in and begin working the muscles. However, it is recommended that you take the time to first properly position your body. You will be working hard to achieve your desired results. You certainly don't want to lose exercise time to nurse an injury! As always, carefully position your body according to the instructions provided when doing any of the following hip and thigh exercises. Locking your knees or placing your feet and legs in an improper position can redirect the stress to the wrong muscles or joints.

Inner-Thigh Wide-Stance Squats

This is almost the same exercise as the regular squat (see page 176), but the wide stance puts more emphasis on the thighs instead of the quadriceps.

Start Position

Assume a wide-leg stance with your feet planted firmly on the floor, with each foot out a little wider than shoulder width. Your feet can be facing out slightly (at a 45-degree angle), but make sure your knees are in line over your big toes. Tuck your abs in and look directly ahead and focus on a point at eye level and continue to focus on it to keep your head and back straight throughout the exercise. Position the unweighted bar across the back of your shoulders and hold it by gripping it on either side so your forearms are straight up and down.

Movement

Slowly lower yourself to a squatting position by bending your legs at the knees. Descend to a position where your thighs are parallel to the ground. Slowly return to the start position. Repeat for three sets of ten repetitions.

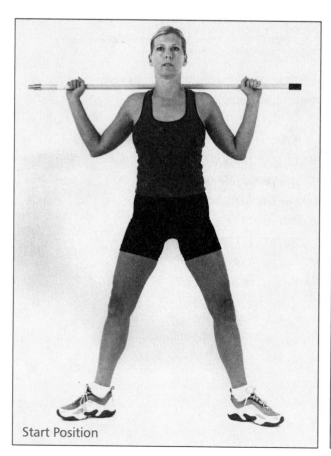

Start Position

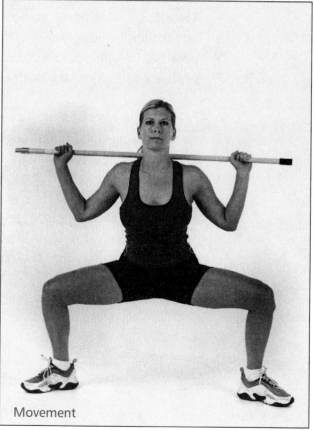

Movement

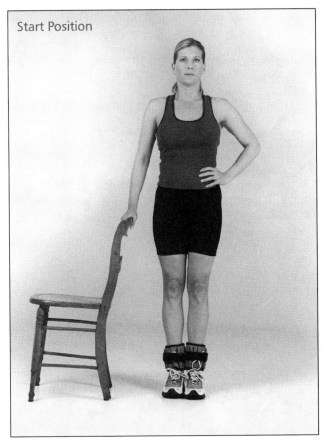

Start Position

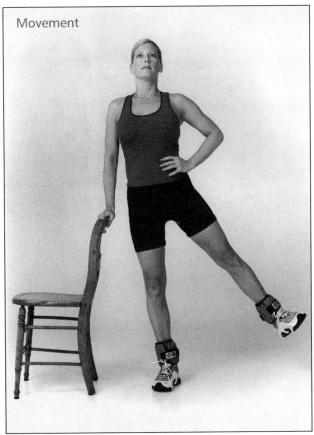

Movement

Standing Leg Lifts with Ankle Weights

■ ■ ■ This exercise works the abductors, or outer thighs.

Start Position
With 1-pound ankle weights on each leg, stand with your feet together next to a chair (or wall), with one hand on the chair for balance. Unlock your knees, tuck in your tummy, and roll back your shoulders.

Movement
Keeping your knee slightly bent, lift the working leg straight out to the side. Your foot should remain flexed. Lift as far as you can without moving your upper body. Hold for three seconds in the up position, then slowly lower your leg to the start position. Repeat for twelve repetitions, then alternate legs. Do a total of three sets. Beginners can do this without the 1-pound ankle weight for the first two weeks. Advanced trainers can use 2 pounders.

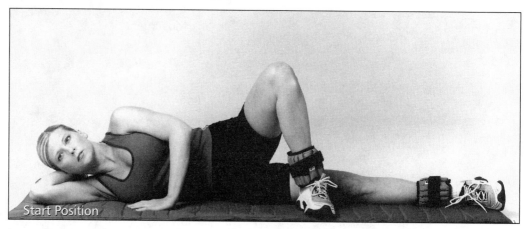

Start Position

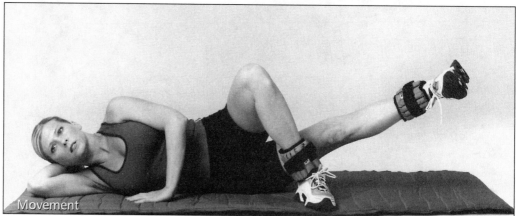

Movement

Inner-Thigh Lifts

This is a difficult movement in the beginning because your thigh muscle is probably weak from not being used. Keep working at it and it will get easier.

Start Position

Lie on your right side on a mat on the floor. Support your upper body by resting on your right arm. Straighten your right leg along the floor. Bend your left knee and place the sole of your left foot on the floor in front of your right leg.

Movement

Keeping your right leg straight, concentrate on using your inner-thigh muscles to raise your right leg off the floor as high as you can. Do not move your upper body. Hold the raised position for three seconds and feel your inner thighs contract. Slowly lower your right leg to the start position on the floor. Repeat for ten repetitions. Switch sides and do ten repetitions for the other leg. Do a total of three sets for each leg.

Side Leg Raises

This exercise works the outer thigh.

Start Position

Lie on your right side on an exercise mat, supporting your upper body by leaning on your right arm. Keep your right leg straight and on the mat during the exercise, or if you need more support, you can bend the right leg. Your left leg should be straight out and resting on top of your right leg.

Movement

Raise your left leg up, creating a slight angle with the floor. Hold for five seconds at the top position and feel your outer thighs contracting. Slowly lower the leg to the start position. Repeat for fifteen repetitions. Alternate sides and do ten repetitions for the right leg. Do a total of three sets for each leg.

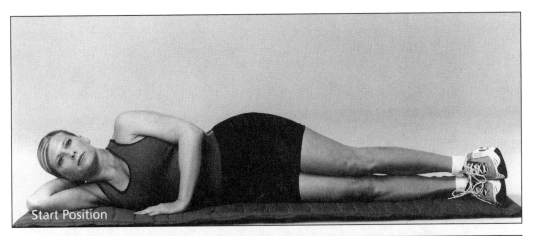

Start Position

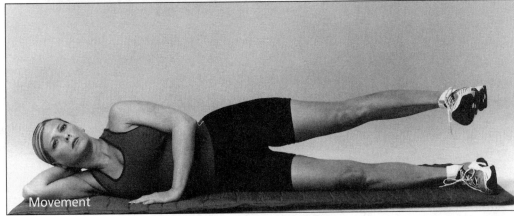

Movement

Scissors

■ ■ ■ This exercise works both the outer and inner thigh.

Start Position Lie on your back on a mat on the floor. Place your palms flat on the floor, under your buttocks. Raise your legs straight up, almost perpendicular to the floor, keeping your knees just slightly unlocked. Turn your knees slightly outward and point your toes out slightly.

Movement Move both legs out as far as possible, keeping your knees just slightly unlocked and your legs at the same slightly out-turned angle. Remember to control the movement and concentrate on the contraction in your inner and outer thighs. Return your legs to the start position but do not cross your feet over as in other scissors movements. Repeat the movement twenty-five times. Work your way up to fifty repetitions, as this is a slightly easy but effective exercise. Do two sets.

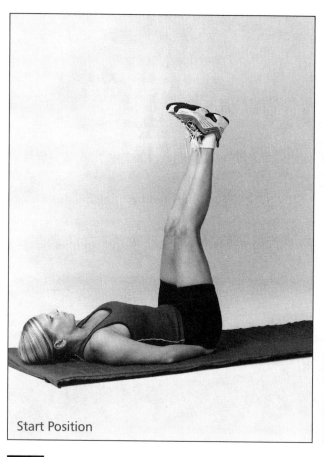

Start Position

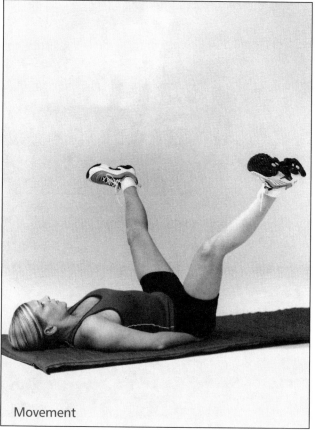

Movement

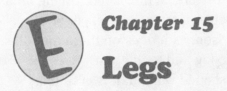

Chapter 15
Legs

Long, lean, shapely legs—who doesn't want them? Working the legs is a very important part of your body-shaping program. Although the legs get plenty of work in daily life activities, you still need to design a program for the legs that will help you sculpt the shape that you want.

Take a Look in the Mirror

How is your body proportioned? What is the proportion of your upper leg to your lower leg? Your upper body to your lower body? Do you have solid thighs and quads but little calves? Think of some men you have seen who work on their upper bodies and neglect their lower bodies, mistakenly thinking that "big biceps" are all they need. Do the broad shoulders, strong back, and muscular arms of your upper body make your lower body look puny in comparison, as it does on these men? If so, then you'll want to work on sculpting and toning your legs.

If you are one of those pear-shaped women, it is even more important to body shape your legs. You will want to tone and change the shape of the upper-leg area and then build up your calf muscles to give balance to the legs as a whole. This will help to get rid of the pear shape and create a well-proportioned and toned body.

Those of you who are fortunate enough to have spent time devoted to certain sports and activities such as tennis, bicycling, dance, swimming, or any other endeavor in which your legs were used, probably already have a natural musculature to build on. On the other hand, it would be easy to understand how in this modern world, one's legs would get virtually no exercise without dedicating specific exercises for that reason. These days it's possible to get through an entire lifetime without having to walk any significant distances.

Why Exercise the Legs?

Let's take a moment to give homage to the legs. Think about all that your legs do for you on a daily basis. They take you where you want to go, they support you as you stand still, they take you away from situations you'd rather avoid, they allow you to jump up and down in excitement, they help you to chase after the kids—the list goes on and on. If you are having difficulty appreciating your legs, think about what life would be like if you were unable to use them.

Now that you have given your legs the respect they deserve, can you think of any reason why you wouldn't want to strengthen and tone the muscles of the legs? Likely not. To give your legs more strength ultimately improves your quality of life. To give your legs more stamina ultimately allows you to enjoy that quality of life for longer periods of time. Giving your legs shape and definition allows you to show them off and improves your self-esteem.

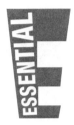

If these reasons aren't enough to give you the motivation needed to exercise your legs, think of the wardrobe you can build with strong and shapely legs. No longer will you have to hide your legs beneath baggy pants. You will be able to buy shorts, skirts, and capris that will show off your results and add a little flair to your outward appearance.

Set Your Goals

So you know you want to sculpt the legs, but what are your goals? Really scrutinize yourself in the mirror. Try to picture yourself at your ideal body shape. If you are planning to create this ideal body shape, how do the legs fit in? Allowing yourself to picture your legs at their ideal shape now will help you to visualize this later as you are doing the exercises.

Do your legs remind you of sticks, barely able to support your body? Perhaps this skinny look doesn't appeal to you or it may make your body look out of proportion. If so, then you will be exercising to build muscle and shape. You will need to concentrate on the muscles being worked as you do the following exercises.

Do your legs seem thick and give your body the overall appearance of being bottom-heavy? Just like the skinny legs, this can make your body seem ill-proportioned. If this is the case, you will want to exercise to make the legs narrower and give a better shape and definition to them.

Anatomy of the Legs

The muscles of the front of the upper leg are called the quadriceps (quads) and the muscles of the back of the upper leg are called the hamstrings or thigh biceps. The quadriceps (quad means four) is a four-part muscle that runs down the front of the thigh to the kneecap. It works when you extend your leg. The hamstrings are the three muscles in the back of the upper leg that work together to flex the knee, rotate the leg, and extend the hips. This muscle group is also sometimes known as the "leg biceps" because the muscle has two heads, similar to the arm biceps muscle.

The calf muscles are the main muscles in the lower leg and are called the gastrocnemius and the soleus. The gastrocnemius works to flex the knee and to flex the foot downward. The soleus is located directly underneath the gastrocnemius. It functions to flex the foot downward, as you do when you push off with each step while walking.

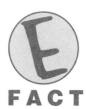

FACT

Knowing the anatomy of the muscles you will be working will help you to visualize their efforts while you are exercising. Visualization helps the mind to concentrate on the task at hand. If you ever thought that exercising requires little to no thought, think again!

Exercises for the Legs

Regardless of what your goals are or how you visualize your ideal body shape, the exercises in this chapter will help you to achieve the results you want. These exercises are simple yet effective and are common to most exercise programs simply because they work.

The great thing about leg exercises is that they not only strengthen and tone the legs, but they also often work to strengthen other areas of the body. You will notice that some of these exercises work the buttock muscles as well. Of course, all require some balance and therefore make the entire body work to maintain that balance.

As you do these exercises, visualize your results and think of all the reasons why strong and toned legs are important to you. This will help you to maintain the motivation and determination needed to achieve the desired results. Now that you're geared up to work the legs, let's get to it!

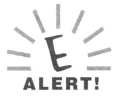

ALERT!

Because your legs are going to be used when working any other area of your body, they are performing double duty when you also work them specifically. This is why it is very important that you do not skimp on the warm-up section of your routine.

Do's and Don'ts

Before beginning the exercises, take a few moments to review some general exercise do's and don'ts:

- **Warm up.** Do light aerobics and stretch before working out to prepare your body for the exercises to come.
- **Follow a routine.** Set aside a quiet place and a regular time for your workout.
- **Take it easy.** Don't overtrain any body part. Avoid injury by "listening" to your body.
- **Visualize.** Concentrate on the muscle being worked—"see it" contract and tighten in your mind's eye.
- **Breathe.** Continue with regular breathing as you work out. Avoid the tendency to hold your breath as you exert yourself.

Just a Reminder

Unless you have very little fat on your legs, exercising the legs to strengthen and tone the muscles is not sufficient to achieve the results you desire. As you know, weight training and resistance exercises will not get rid of the layer of fat covering the muscle. You will need to incorporate an aerobics regimen and healthy diet into your body shaping plan if you want to be able to see the results of the hard work you've done to tone those leg muscles.

Squats with Unweighted Bar

• • ▪ This exercise works the quads and the buttocks.

Start Position

Stand with your feet shoulder-width apart and place an unweighted bar across the back of your shoulders. Place your hands on the bar in a comfortable position. Tuck in your abs and roll your shoulders back. Focus on looking at a point directly in front of you to help you keep your head and back straight during the movement.

Movement

Slowly lower yourself into a squatting position by bending your legs at the knees. As you bend, be careful to keep your knees in a direct line above your feet. Concentrating on the contraction in your quads and buttocks and keeping your abs tucked in, bend your knees until your thighs are almost parallel to the floor without compromising your form and then slowly return to the start position. Repeat ten times for three sets.

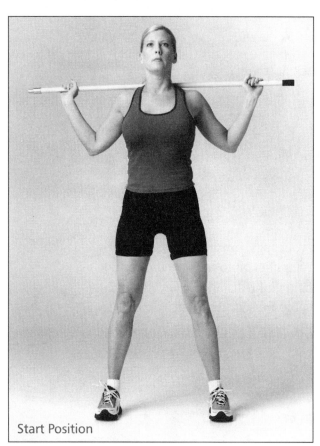

Start Position

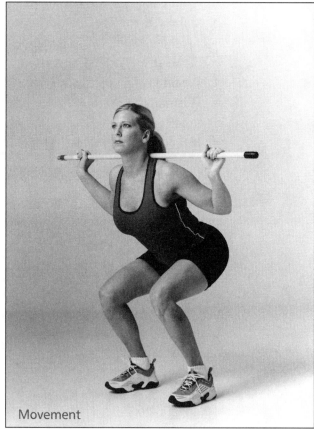

Movement

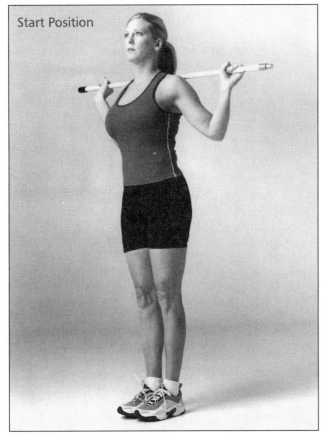

Start Position

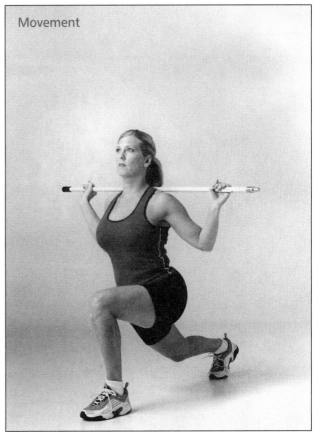

Movement

Lunges with Unweighted Bar

■ ■ ■   This exercise works the quads and glutes.

Start Position   Stand with your feet shoulder-width apart and place an unweighted bar across the backs of your shoulders. Grasp the bar in a comfortable position. Focus on looking at a point directly in front of you to help you keep your head and back straight during the movement.

Movement   Step forward with your left foot as far as possible, bending your right knee as you do so. Concentrate on keeping your torso upright and not leaning forward with it into the movement. You may feel the stretch in your quadriceps muscles and a contraction in the buttock muscles. Step into the lunge bending your front knee until your thigh is almost parallel to the ground. Your knee should not extend beyond your big toe. Try to keep it above your ankle. Do three sets of ten repetitions for each leg.

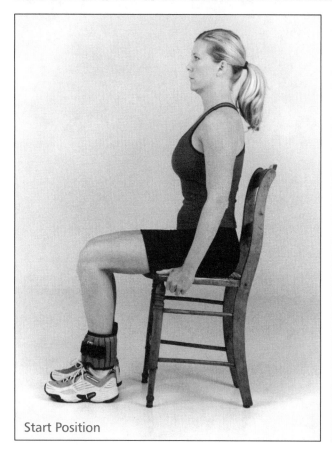

Start Position

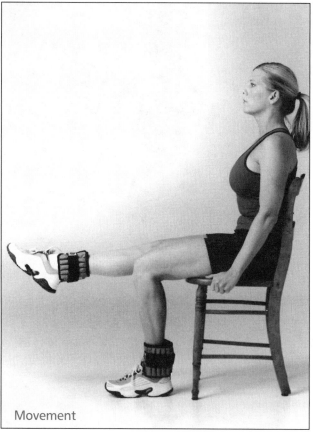

Movement

Leg Extensions with Ankle Weights

This exercise works the quads.

Start Position Sit on an exercise bench or chair. Place ankle weights on each leg. Spread your legs so they are about hip-width apart, keeping your knees in a line with your feet. Tuck your abs in and hold on to the sides of the chair or bench.

Movement Extend one leg forward and up without locking your knee. Hold for three seconds and feel the contraction in your quads. Slowly lower the leg to the start position except do not allow it to touch the floor. Repeat the extension ten times. Switch to the other leg and repeat for ten repetitions with that leg. Do three sets for each leg.

Leg Curls with Ankle Weights

▪ ▪ ▪ This exercise works the hamstrings.

Start Position Kneel on the floor in an all-fours position with an ankle weight on each leg. Place your elbows on the floor under your shoulders. Keep your back straight and avoid dropping your head. Extend one leg back with the heel in line with the buttocks.

Movement Raise the extended leg up horizontal to the floor and then curl it by pulling your heel toward your buttocks. Slowly uncurl your leg and lower to the start position. Repeat ten times then switch to the other leg for another ten repetitions. Do three sets for each leg.

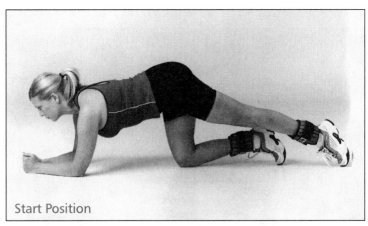

Start Position

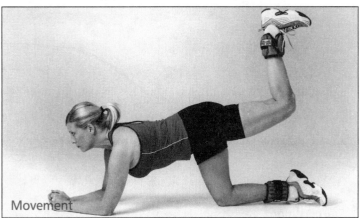

Movement

Standing Toe Raises

For this exercise, you will need to purchase a piece of wood that is about 4 to 5 feet long and 3 to 4 inches thick. This exercise will work the calf muscles.

Start Position

Stand on the block of wood with your feet together. Slowly slide your feet back so that only the ball of each foot and your toes are still on the wood and the rest of the foot is hanging off. Stand straight, roll your shoulders back, and tuck your tummy in. Hold onto a chair for support and balance. Lift the foot of the nonworking leg up toward your buttocks.

Movement

Slowly lower the heel of your working leg toward the floor just about touching it but not quite. Feel the stretch in the calf muscle. Then slowly raise your heel upward until it is lifted all the way up, higher than the ball of your foot, and your toes are pressing against the wood block. Slowly lower your heel again and repeat the movement ten times for three sets of ten repetitions for each leg.

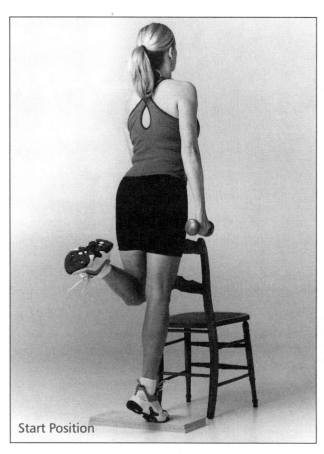

Start Position

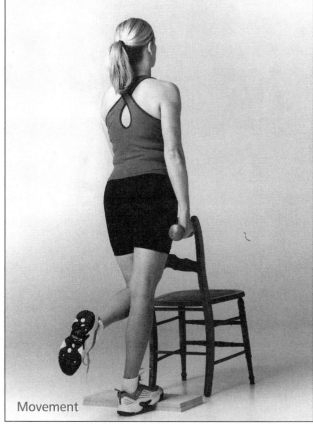

Movement

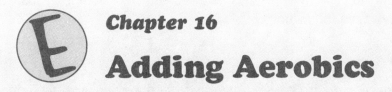

Chapter 16

Adding Aerobics

As we discussed in earlier chapters, it will be important to add an aerobic component to your body-shaping program. You will need to lower the amount of body fat covering the muscles so that you can reveal the toned and shaped muscle underneath. So, now it is time to get started with the aerobic portion of your program.

Benefits of Aerobic Exercise

Simply put, aerobic exercise works this way: As you exert yourself, your body demands an increased supply of oxygen to make energy. As you breathe, the oxygen goes from your lungs into your bloodstream. From there, your heart pumps it to your muscles, and the oxygen is used to break down carbohydrates, fats, and proteins into the energy that your muscles need to function.

Burn Fat

Aerobic exercise goes a long way toward melting away fat. It increases your metabolism and when done frequently and regularly enough, may actually increase your metabolic rate—the rate at which you burn calories as you go about your day-to-day activities. The more you do aerobics, the more your aerobic fitness level increases and the more your heart, lungs, and muscles become more efficient at doing their job of burning fat. It is inevitable that you will get leaner and see a significant loss of weight and fat if you perform this component of your program faithfully.

Feel Good

Looking good isn't the only benefit of adding aerobic exercise to your body-shaping plan. You will feel better, too. Many people swear that regular aerobic exercise has lifted depression, cured them of sleepless-ness, and generally improved their overall mood. Exercise experts say that this feeling of general well-being that results from regular exercise is a biochemical reality. It is said that during and after exercise your brain releases endorphins, chemical substances that are associated with pleasure. Athletes refer to this as the "endorphin high."

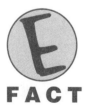

FACT

If you are a smoker, aerobic exercise may not appeal to you, since you will likely have a harder time getting the air you need. However, if you wish to quit smoking, aerobic exercise can help. Studies have shown that aerobic exercise actually curbs the cravings as well as improves lung function.

Improve Your Health

Aerobic exercise improves your general health as well. Because it strengthens the heart and lungs, you are less susceptible to heart and lung diseases. It reduces your risk of heart disease, diabetes, and vascular disease. The cardiovascular system will work more efficiently and become more durable if an aerobic activity is performed regularly. This in turn promotes longer living. But this benefit carries even further. Not only may you live longer, but you'll also have more energy to live a fuller life!

How Much and How Long

How much is enough? A general consensus is that you need to work a minimum of thirty minutes a session for at least three to five sessions a week. Opinions on this differ but all agree that the more you do, the better your results will be. Ideally, you will want to maintain 65 to 85 percent of your maximum heart rate for fifteen to twenty minutes during each aerobic exercise session. By doing aerobics for thirty minutes, this allows some time to get your heart rate up to its efficiency level as well as some time at the end to cool down.

Determining Your Heart Rate

There are a couple of different formulas you can use to calculate your heart rate to make sure you are working at a level of effectiveness. Either of these formulas can be used to find your maximum heart rate. Once you have your maximum heart rate, take 65 to 85 percent of that to find your ideal training range. The first formula simply subtracts your age from 220. For instance, if you are thirty-five, then your maximum heart rate is 185 beats per minute, with a training range of 120 to 157 beats per minute. The second, more recent formula calculates your maximum heart rate by multiplying your age by 0.7 and then subtracting that from 208. Again, let's say you are thirty-five years old. With this formula, your maximum heart rate is 184 beats per minute, with a training range of 120 to 157 beats per minute. As you can see, these two formulas produce very similar results, so you can use either to come up with a target heart rate.

Using the ideal training heart rate can help you to determine whether you are working hard enough to achieve results. However, if you are new to aerobic activity, it is probably enough for a while just to make sure you are working hard. An easier way to evaluate your level of intensity is to simply ask yourself how much longer you can carry on the activity you are currently doing. You should be working hard enough that you could not conceive of going on for hours but not so hard that you need to stop right away.

Start Slow

Start out slowly. If it has been a long time since you have done aerobic exercise or if you are a beginner, remember to start slowly. Don't be discouraged if at first all you can manage are ten-minute sessions. Gradually increase your time by adding five minutes every few sessions and before a few weeks are done, you will have reached the thirty-minute minimum for a session. Remember that you are not racing anyone and this is not a competition. The only one measuring your progress is yourself, and you can afford to give yourself time to do this right.

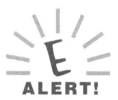
ALERT!

If you reach a point during your aerobic exercise when you think you are too tired to go on, don't stop moving. Stopping suddenly can cause your muscles to cramp up and may even cause you to become dizzy. Instead, march in place for a few moments to allow your body time to adjust to the cool down without stopping completely.

Aerobic Activities

What kind of aerobic activity should you choose? There is no one answer to this question. You should choose the one that you enjoy doing. If walking is appealing to you, then upgrade your daily walk into a "power walk." Gradually increase the speed and distance you are doing and put some force into your stride. After a while, add light hand weights to your routine.

If you are lucky enough to belong to a gym, put the aerobic machines to good use. There is a wide array of choices at every gym: treadmills, bicycles, rowing machines, stair climbers, spinning classes, step classes, hip-hop aerobics, and endless varieties of other classes.

A Home Treadmill

A home treadmill can provide you with a year-round opportunity to exercise, and they are not as boring as you might think. There are many models available to choose from, ranging from basic to deluxe, depending on the amount of money you can spare to spend. Though it may seem like a lot at first blush, a home treadmill is a smart investment that will last a long time. Another benefit to having your own treadmill is that those old excuses about not having time to go to the gym don't work anymore!

Owning your own treadmill has several benefits. First and foremost is the benefit of convenience. No longer do you have to make the commute to and from the gym to get a good aerobic workout. Also, you needn't worry anymore about the weather, the mean dog down the street, or gawking passersby. You can walk, run, or jog in the comfort of your own home.

Another benefit to having a home treadmill is that you can set a program and remain consistent. For example, many treadmills have programs that can be set at various intensities. Some of these programs will include varying speeds and differing inclines to give your body a great overall workout. By using a treadmill, you bypass obstacles you would face in walking/running outdoors such as street crossings, pedestrians, potholes, and strong winds.

Another great benefit to owning a treadmill is that you can prevent boredom. You can set up a television in front of the treadmill and catch up on your favorite programs while working out. Most televisions have an outlet for earplugs or headphones so you can hear the voices of the television over the noise of the treadmill. Most electronics stores sell headphones with 15- or 25-foot cords so you can be quite a distance from the television, move around freely on the treadmill, and still be plugged in. Many treadmills also offer a stand on which you can place a book or magazine. Of course, you can also play upbeat music that will help to get you in the mood for a vigorous workout. Anything you can use to help prevent boredom will aid your workout tremendously.

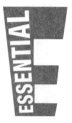

If you are not an outdoors type and you cannot afford a gym, consider purchasing exercise videotapes or DVDs. There are numerous wonderful exercise videotapes to choose from, and you can do any program from Pilates to kickboxing in the privacy of your own home.

Choose an Activity or Two

The wonderful thing about aerobic activities is that you have a variety of types to choose from. Since you are going to participate in an aerobic activity at least three times a week, it's best if you can find something that you enjoy doing. The more you enjoy an activity, the more likely you will be to remain consistent in performing that activity. Of course, you needn't choose just one; you can always vary your workout by alternating between a few different activities. Remember, variety is the spice of life!

The following is a list of aerobic activities you can choose from:

- Walking/power walking
- Jogging
- Cycling
- Hiking
- Swimming
- Water aerobics
- Treadmill training
- Exercise classes
- Step aerobics
- Kickboxing
- Dancing
- Cross-country skiing
- Spinning
- Tennis

- Racquetball/squash
- Inline skating
- Jumping rope
- Rowing

These are just a few suggestions to get you started. If you find another activity that gets your heart rate up and can be sustained for approximately thirty minutes a session, then great! Add that activity to the aerobic portion of your body-shaping plan. Nowhere is it stated that exercising has to be void of all fun.

Vary Your Workout

Some fitness enthusiasts say that it is important to vary your workout routine so that your body does not become accustomed to the same movements performed every time and thus build up a sort of tolerance to them. Some disagree and state that your body is incapable of building up a tolerance. It's up to you which argument you believe, and you can plan your body-shaping routine accordingly. However, there are some perks to varying your routine regardless of whether or not you believe your body will build up a tolerance.

Best Investment of Time

Your aerobics workout is going to cost you time (of course, this is time well spent, but time nonetheless). Unless you have nothing at all else to do, time is going to be a concern. Although there is no way to cut the time needed for a good aerobic workout, there is a way to make sure you get the best investment for your time spent.

By adding short bursts of higher-intensity training, you take your aerobic exercise up a notch and even lose weight faster. For instance, let's say you have chosen to incorporate a jogging schedule as the aerobic part of your body-shaping plan. You have figured out your maximum heart rate and thus your training heart rate. You plan to keep up a pace that will fall within the training heart rate range for twenty minutes. While this is an excellent plan, you can take it up a notch by incorporating short bursts of sprints that will take your heart rate up to the higher end of the training heart rate range or even beyond it. By doing this, you will be getting more aerobic benefits for the time spent.

For those of you just beginning aerobic exercises, figuring your training heart rate range isn't necessary. But this doesn't mean you cannot throw in spurts of higher-intensity activities. For example, let's say that you have chosen walking as your preferred form of aerobic activity. You can add intervals of higher intensity by jogging for a few minutes and then go back to walking. The more intervals of jogging you can incorporate, the better.

This not only helps to build stamina and burn the fat faster. Studies show that varying the intensity levels of an aerobic activity allows the benefits (such as higher metabolic rates) to carry on longer following the exercise period. In fact, one study found that during the twenty-four hours following a run interspersed with sprints, runners had a metabolic rate that was 5 to 10 percent higher than that of people who run at a steady pace.

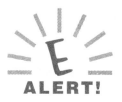

ALERT!

Don't try to start out with more than you can handle. If you are just beginning to exercise, you shouldn't expect to be able to run for a half-hour straight. It's best to begin slowly. Start with walking and then work your way up to jogging. Eventually, you will be able to run the entire thirty minutes.

Prevent Boredom

Another good reason to vary your workout is to prevent boredom. If you are a walker, try a different route once in a while. If you love the treadmill, vary your routine by listening to different music, adding arm movements, adding hand weights, and by not doing the same programmed routine every time. Most treadmills come with at least four or five different programmed routines, some more difficult than others. If you go to the gym, use the pool and swim laps a few times a week in place of machine work. There are workouts designed to be done in water—find out what they are and try them. Join the water aerobics class—it is fun and if you are not coordinated, this is the class for you because nobody can see you swinging the wrong leg under water!

It is important that you maintain a high level of motivation. Aerobic exercise isn't always easy, but that doesn't mean it shouldn't be fun. If you incorporate an activity or activities that you enjoy doing, you are much more likely to stick with your workout schedule.

What to Wear

If you are shopping for what to wear as you begin your body-shaping program, you may become intimidated by all the products available. First of all, there is no reason why you should spend loads of money on workout clothing (unless you have it to spend and want to). This body-shaping program is meant to be cost-effective, and that includes clothing. However, there are a couple of things you'll want to keep in mind as you're shopping.

Shop for Comfort

Shop for comfort, not for style. This is where many people mess up. Most want to be able to look great in those tight workout getups. This might entice you to buy them, but once taken off the hanger and put on, they all of a sudden seem less than glamorous. Of all things, clothing should be the last thing to discourage you from working out.

Wear loose and comfortable clothing so that your movements are not restricted and choose "breathable" fabrics such as cotton or synthetic and cotton blends that are designed to wick the sweat away from your body.

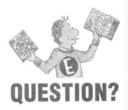

QUESTION?

Should I buy clothes that are a couple sizes too small to help motivate me to fit into them?
It isn't recommended that you shop for clothes that will fit your ideal body shape until you have actually reached that ideal body shape. Doing so may prove to depress you rather than motivate you. Use the shopping trip as a reward for all of your hard work once you have achieved your goals.

If you are a woman, then a good exercise bra is a must to support your breasts during active movements. Try a few different types to ensure you get the right fit and the style that works best for you. If you are a plus-size woman, take heart because now more than ever before there is a wide range of exercise clothes made just for you. If your local stores do not carry what you need, do some research on the Internet and you are sure to find your size available on a number of Web sites. Select clothing that feels good and is appropriate for whatever activity you have chosen.

Footwear

Proper footwear is especially important. Buy a good pair of athletic sneakers. This is a purchase that you do not want to skimp on, because stability and comfort are essential for a successful aerobic workout. For optimal comfort, you need shoes that properly fit the length and width of your feet. Have your feet measured every time you buy new athletic shoes, as the size of your feet changes as you age. Also remember that your feet swell when you work out, so you don't want shoes that are tight when you try them on at the store.

Look for shoes that are made of a flexible material that breathes, such as mesh, and that have sufficient arch support and cushioning. Enlist the aid of a knowledgeable shoe salesperson to help you pick out a good pair and to check how they fit your feet. Walk around or even jog in place with the shoes on to make sure they aren't too tight or too loose. Your toes shouldn't feel pinched and your feet shouldn't slide around in the shoes.

It is also important to check the wear of your shoes every so often. Examine the soles in particular, looking for any spots that are worn or uneven, especially around the edges. If you notice any unevenness to the soles of your shoes, buy a new pair. You'll be surprised just how quickly your shoes will wear out when you work out regularly. (E)

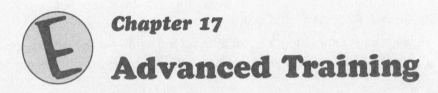

Chapter 17

Advanced Training

If you have achieved the goals you set earlier, you may be ready to take your body-shaping regimen a step further with advanced training. This chapter will cover advanced training techniques that you may want to try to help you set and reach new goals. Keep in mind, this is only for those who have already completed a beginner's body-shaping program.

Ready for the Next Step

If you have been following your personal body-shaping plan faithfully for a period of time, you will know that certain changes have taken place in your body. It is likely that you have experienced changes to your mood, strength, health, weight, attitude, measurements, the way you wear you clothes, and even the clothes you choose to wear. You may have experienced changes for the better in your sleep patterns, and changes in your productivity level at work and home. By now, you are probably sold on the advantages of the body-shaping lifestyle and ready for the next step in your training.

Full Body Program

If your basic personalized program consisted of targeted exercises for few select body parts that you wanted to improve along with the aerobic or cardio portion, you can always go to another level by adding more body parts and enlarging the scope of your program to a full body program. When you add more body parts to your basic program, you might want to reduce the amount of exercises you do for each body part down to two. This book presents at least four exercises for each body part. If you are focusing on a particular part of your body, you will want to do all four exercises.

Alternate Workout Days

One way to advance your workout to another level is to alternate workout days so that on one day you are focusing on specific parts and the next day you are doing an overall total body program. For example, if abs and arms are your two trouble spots but you want to expand your workout to include the rest of your body, your exercise program might look like this:

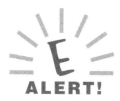

It is always important to stretch some after your workout because that is when your muscles are warm and pliable, and you get the best stretch and lengthening effect.

Monday, Wednesday, Friday

- 5 minutes of warm-up stretch
- 20 minutes on treadmill
- Standing Alternate Biceps Curls with Dumbbells (3 sets of 10 reps)
- Dumbbell Kick-Backs (3 sets of 10 reps)
- Seated Two-Arm Triceps Extensions (2 sets of 10 reps)
- Seated Concentration Curls (2 sets of 10 reps)
- Classic Crunches (2 sets of 15 reps)
- Knee-Up Leg Raises (2 sets of 15 reps)
- Oblique Crunches (2 sets of 15 reps)
- 5 minutes of cool-down stretch

Tuesday, Thursday, Saturday (Sunday off)

- 5 minutes of warm-up stretch
- 20-minute power walk outside
- *Chest:* Dumbbell Presses on a Bench or Mat (3 sets of 10 reps)
- *Shoulders:* Lateral Raises with Dumbbells (3 sets of 10 reps)
- *Biceps:* Standing Alternate Biceps Curls with Dumbbells (3 sets of 10 reps)
- *Triceps:* Seated Two-Arm Triceps Extensions (3 sets of 10 reps)
- *Back:* Bent-Over Rowing with Unweighted Bar (3 sets of 10 reps)
- *Legs:* Squats with Unweighted Bar (3 sets of 10 reps)
- *Hips and thighs:* Inner-Thigh Wide-Stance Squats (3 sets of 10 reps) and Standing Leg Lifts with Ankle Weights (3 sets of 10 reps)
- *Calves:* Standing Toe Raises (2 sets of 15 reps)
- *Abs:* Classic Crunches (2 sets of 15 reps)
- 5 minutes of cool-down stretch

The previous is just a suggested sample of one type of program you can set up, but the variations are endless. You should set up the program that works best for you and is tailored to your particular needs, likes, and dislikes.

Another good way to increase the effectiveness of our workout is to apply some of the advanced training principles that the serious bodybuilders use. A few of these will be discussed here along with a description of how you can adapt them to your body-shaping program.

Straight Sets

Before we discuss some of the advanced techniques, first you need a label for the type of exercises you have been performing up to now. If you have followed the instructions in the body part chapters, you have been performing what are known as "straight sets." Straight sets are defined as a series of repetitions of a particular exercise, repeated for a number of times, with pauses of 60 to 90 seconds in between each series, or set. So when you do three sets of ten repetitions of biceps curls, you are performing straight sets. Generally, it is advisable to perform at least two or three sets of each exercise. Also, if you choose to do more than one exercise for a specific body part, then you would always perform them together, before moving on to perform an exercise for another body part. Now we can move on to more advanced training techniques.

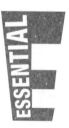

Even though you feel you are ready for advanced training techniques, don't forget about the straight sets. The advanced training techniques outlined here are for irregular use and should be used along with the straight sets you have been performing.

Pyramid Sets

One of the easiest advanced-training principles for you to adapt is known as the *pyramid technique*. We already know that weight training is an exercise method that uses the principle of progressive resistance. That is, you help your muscles to grow by using them, and then using them some more with added weight to add resistance, and then gradually increasing that weight as your muscle grows to adapt to the change. With pyramid training, you are applying this principle in one set of exercises, in one training session, instead of over a period of time.

Example Pyramid Technique

It works like this: Say you have been performing straight sets of lateral raises for the shoulders as suggested in the earlier chapter: three sets of ten repetitions with 5-pound dumbbells. You have been doing this for four weeks and have progressed to a higher weight, so now you are doing straight sets with a heavier weight: three sets of ten repetitions with 8-pound dumbbells. If you want to apply the pyramid-training principle in order to kick things up a notch, your exercise instruction would look like this:

1. One set of twelve repetitions with 5-pound dumbbells
2. One set of ten repetitions with 8-pound dumbbells
3. One set of eight repetitions with 10-pound dumbbells

If you take a look at the previous instruction you will see that with each set you are increasing the weight but decreasing the amount of reps you are performing. You are pyramiding up with the weight and down with the reps. This technique stimulates muscle development for a few reasons. One is that you are increasing the resistance within a short amount of time and forcing the muscle to work harder. Secondly, you are varying the resistance and reps used and that "surprises" the muscle that might have become used to the regular work of three sets of ten at a stable weight over a period of time. The variety serves the purpose of not letting the muscle get a chance to become adjusted to the exercise.

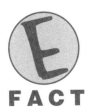

FACT

Many fitness enthusiasts live by the theory that you need to surprise your muscles to get the greatest results. This involves mixing up your routine so that your muscles don't know what is coming.

When to Avoid Pyramiding

You can apply this principle to almost any of the exercises described in this book. The only ones that pyramiding cannot be used with are the exercises that do not use weights to add resistance, such as the crunches for the abs. Many advanced trainers do hold a 5- or 10-pound weight plate across their chest with their hands crossed over it while performing crunches and this does add resistance, but the use of any plates heavier than that would not be feasible, so this is an example of an exercise where pyramiding cannot be applied.

The Next Pyramid Level

When you are attempting to use this technique, do not be distressed if at first you have a difficult time with the last set at the highest weight. If you are doing this right, you should strain with the last set because you should be using a weight that is not easy for you. The weight you are used to should be either the base of the pyramid (the first set) or the middle of the pyramid (the second set). The third set should always be performed with a weight that is new and a challenge to your muscles. After your muscles get adjusted to the first pyramid you use, then you would graduate to the next level. Using the same example as before, the lateral raise, the next pyramid would look like this:

1. One set of twelve repetitions with 8-pound weights
2. One set of ten repetitions with 10-pound weights
3. One set of eight (or six at first) repetitions with 12-pound weights

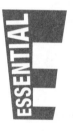

Using pyramid sets not only works to give your muscles that added "oomph," but is also a great way to add some variety to your workout. If you find that you've become bored with the same old routine, by all means, mix it up a bit!

Reverse Pyramid Sets

One reason to apply advanced techniques is to get off a plateau or to increase the amount of change you are seeing in a body part. For more variety, try this variation of the pyramid technique.

The reverse pyramid is when you start with the heaviest weight first, and then progress to the lighter weight with the increased reps. Picture a standard pyramid with the exercise description applied to it as follows: The base of the pyramid is your first set of many reps with light weight, the middle of the pyramid is your second set with less reps, and the top of the pyramid is your third set with the least amount of reps.

Then, picture the pyramid in reverse, with the base on top, and see how the exercise movements have been reversed. The base of the pyramid is now the narrowest part, so your first set would be the least amount of reps; your second set would be a few more reps; and the third set would be the most amount of reps because the widest part is now at the top.

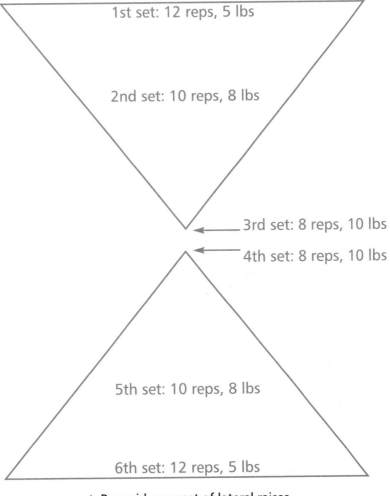

1st set: 12 reps, 5 lbs

2nd set: 10 reps, 8 lbs

3rd set: 8 reps, 10 lbs

4th set: 8 reps, 10 lbs

5th set: 10 reps, 8 lbs

6th set: 12 reps, 5 lbs

▲ Pyramid superset of lateral raises

With the reverse pyramid, you are varying your workout again by not only changing the weight and reps used with each set, but by reversing the order in which it is done, heaviest to lightest, instead of vice versa.

When you really want to bomb a particular body part, do a superset of both pyramids for that body part, and then follow it up with a reverse pyramid for another exercise for the same body part. (Supersets will be explained next, but here it means two exercises for one body part performed one after another with no rest in between.) That program would look like this:

Lateral Raises with Dumbbells—Pyramid Up
1. One set of twelve reps, 5 pounds
2. One set of ten reps, 8 pounds
3. One set of twelve reps, 10 pounds

This is immediately followed by:

Lateral Raises with Dumbbells—Pyramid Down
1. One set of twelve reps, 10 pounds
2. One set of ten reps, 8 pounds
3. One set of eight reps, 5 pounds

This is immediately followed by:

Shoulder Presses with Dumbbells—Pyramid Up
1. One set of twelve reps, 5 pounds
2. One set of ten reps, 8 pounds
3. One set of eight reps, 10 pounds

And this is immediately followed by:

Shoulder Presses with Dumbbells—Pyramid Down
1. One set of eight reps, 10 pounds
2. One set of ten reps, 8 pounds
3. One set of twelve reps, 5 pounds

You have just bombed your shoulders! This is a very advanced technique and you should be very comfortable with your movements and the amount of weight you are working with before attempting this sequence. You can do this with any body part by selecting two exercises for the same body part and then applying the principle of pyramiding up and down and performing the two exercises with very little rest in between.

Supersets

This brings us to a discussion of the next advanced-training technique you can use. Supersets are called such because it is the combining of two exercises for a special effect. One kind of superset is to perform two different exercises for the same muscle together (as is described previously with lateral raises and shoulder presses put together for the shoulders—that is a pyramid superset). Another kind of superset is to perform two different exercises for opposing muscles together.

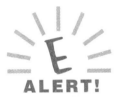

ALERT!

Any of these advanced techniques should be used irregularly. If you were to use these techniques on a regular basis, your muscles run the risk of being overworked and possibly even injured.

Supersets for the Same Body Part

When you are supersetting the same muscle or body part, you alternate sets of one exercise with sets of another for the same muscle. Here is an example of a superset workout for the chest:

1. Dumbbell Presses on a Bench or Mat, one set of ten reps, 5 pounds
2. Dumbbell Chest Flyes, one set of ten reps, 5 pounds
3. Dumbbell Presses, one set of ten reps, 5 pounds
4. Dumbbell Chest Flyes, one set of ten reps, 5 pounds
5. Dumbbell Presses, one set of ten reps, 5 pounds
6. Dumbbell Chest Flyes, one set of ten reps, 5 pounds

Perform these sets in close succession with only a few seconds of rest in between.

Supersets for Opposing Body Parts

When you superset different or opposing muscles or body parts, you are putting together two exercises for different body parts for a special effect. Before we describe the technique, take a look at a list of some suggested opposing muscle groups to work together:

- Biceps and triceps
- Chest and back
- Hips and thighs and buttocks
- Shoulders and arms
- Abs and back
- Chest and shoulders

You can play around with the combinations—the idea is to pick two different but close body parts. The important thing to remember is that you are alternating two exercises rapidly, without much rest in between. Supersets will add variety to your routine and shock your muscles into new growth. Do not perform them on a regular basis; instead, throw them into your routine once in a while to shake things up a bit!

The following is an example of a superset for the chest and shoulders:

1. Alternate Forward Raises with Dumbbells: one set of ten reps with 5-pound dumbbells
2. Shoulder Presses with Dumbbells: one set of ten reps with 5 pounds
3. Alternate Forward Raises with Dumbbells: one set of ten reps with 5-pound dumbbells
4. Shoulder Presses with Dumbbells: one set of ten reps with 5 pounds
5. Alternate Forward Raises with Dumbbells: one set of ten reps with 5-pound dumbbells
6. Shoulder Presses with Dumbbells: one set of ten reps with 5 pounds

Remember to pause only for a few seconds in between sets. You have just performed a superset for the shoulders and chest!

Peak Contraction

Another technique that can boost your workout results is one in which your mind is as important as your strength. In this technique, you will be concentrating very closely on your muscles during the exercise movement. You want to use visualization to isolate the muscle you are working and see it growing and straining to perform the movement. As you are concentrating on the muscle, you will be conscious of the point at which it is at its peak contraction, and you will give your muscle an extra "squeeze" at this point in the movement each time it occurs. *Peak contraction* is defined as the most strenuous point of the exercise; usually this occurs toward the midpoint of any movement. For example, if you are doing a biceps curl, the moment of peak contraction occurs as you are raising your arms up and you reach the point at which you cannot raise them any further. Now, before you start to lower the weight, this is exactly the moment of peak contraction and when you should "squeeze" the muscle.

Using Visualization

The process of using visualization at peak contraction would go like this: As you begin the exercise and raise your arms, you should picture the muscle in your mind and watch it working to perform the movement. At the moment of peak contraction, you will "squeeze" the muscle as hard as you can and hold that squeeze as you pause at the top of the movement. Then, as you release the squeeze, you start to lower the weight. As you return the arm to its start position to begin the exercise movement again, you will visualize the muscle slowly releasing the tension and working lightly to lower the weight.

Proper Body Positioning

This technique requires intense concentration throughout the entire set. Your mind is isolating the muscle and concentrating on it for the entire time. Be careful that you don't concentrate so hard that you forget to breathe and maintain your proper body posture. After working out regularly for a period of time, things like proper body positioning and breathing should become second nature to you if you have been careful in the early stages to remain conscious of doing the exercises properly.

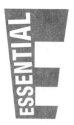

If you have chosen to incorporate one or two of these advanced techniques into your body-shaping plan, take a moment to congratulate yourself for taking your physical well-being to the next level. You have worked hard to achieve this level. You certainly deserve to treat yourself!

Let's review these factors quickly: Correct positioning involves keeping your shoulders rolled back, your head and spine straight, your tummy tucked in, and your elbow and knee joints slightly unlocked, or bent. Proper breathing means that you should breathe in and out regularly being careful that you do not hold your breath. Sometimes during strenuous exercise the natural tendency is to hold your breath, so proper breathing might take some conscious effort.

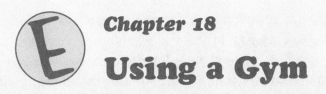

Chapter 18

Using a Gym

W hile many people do their body-shaping program at home, some people choose to utilize their local gyms. Whether you want to take your workout up a notch, meet others who share the same body-shaping interests, or simply want to try your workout in a new environment, the gym can be a great place to put your plan to work.

Advantages of Utilizing a Gym

As you know, the exercises in the body-shaping program as outlined in this book have been designed so that they can easily be done in the comfort of your own home and do not require any high-tech fancy equipment. The program here will work even for those who never step foot inside a gym. However, this isn't to say that you must never work out in a gym. Perhaps you already have a gym membership or working out alone is beginning to bore you. Maybe you want to turn your body-shaping routine up a notch. There are a hundred reasons why you may want to join a gym. Whatever your reason, working out in a gym offers a few advantages over working out at home.

A Fully Equipped Free-Weight Section

The biggest advantage to working out in a gym is probably the fully equipped free-weight section and the availability of machines. Every gym has a free-weight section with a selection of benches, including flat and preset incline and decline benches. Also included in this section are preset dumbbells in nearly any weight you would want (usually 1 to 25 pounds), a preweighted bar at a fixed weight of 45 pounds, and a full rack of weighted plates (usually ½ pound to 50 pounds) to add to the bars. Free-weight sections even include specialized bars designed for particular exercises. For instance, one popular specialized bar is the curling bar, which is designed specifically for doing biceps curls.

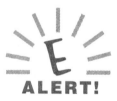

ALERT!

Beware of the gym "chickies." Don't be intimidated by the women with perfect bodies in the revealing spandex tights and sports bras—you are there to do your own business and leave, not to participate in a fashion show.

Using the free-weight section of a gym allows you to intensify your workout at any time. While this body-shaping program doesn't require you to use weights for the most part, it's good to know you have that option once your body becomes accustomed to working out without weights. For anyone interested in challenging his or her body beyond the scope of this body-shaping program or who wants to add resistance to those exercises offered here, the free-weight section of a gym offers a variety of alternatives.

Circuit of Exercise Machines

In addition to the fully equipped free-weight section, every gym has a circuit of exercise machines, including both variable resistance and universal machines. Both universal and variable resistance weight machines position your body to perform a movement that targets specific muscles. The machine supports your body and holds it stationary while it only permits the working muscle to move. (Later in this chapter, we will examine the differences between free-weight training and machine training, offering the pros and cons of each.)

Universal machines use stacks of weight plates with a pin that is moved to vary the weight resistance of the movement. Variable resistance machines use air pressure pumped through a piston to create resistance instead of using a fixed stack of weights. The first popular variable resistance machines were called "Nautilus" machines. Because they were the first and became widely popular in the 1970s, sometimes the term "Nautilus" is misused as the generic term to refer to the entire class of variable resistance machines. One of the advantages of the Nautilus type of machine is that the resistance is applied evenly throughout the full range of motion of the movement.

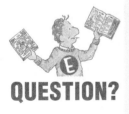

QUESTION?

In what order should I use the machines?
Usually the machines are set up in a "circuit." For instance, you're likely to see the machines set up for the upper body in one section—chest, shoulders, back, biceps, triceps, abs—and then lower body—leg extension, leg biceps, leg press, abductor, adductor, and calf.

The exercise machines offered in most gyms can give your body a great workout when used properly. By following the instructions for each machine, you are able to position your body in a way that targets certain muscles without putting undue stress on other areas of your body. Also, because you are able to control the weight or resistance for each machine, you are in charge of the intensity of your workout. Using these machines helps you to build muscle endurance and strength.

Floor-to-Ceiling Mirrors

Nearly every gym will have its walls set up with floor-to-ceiling mirrors so you can watch yourself work out. No, these mirrors weren't designed to indulge those who are in love with their images. The mirrors serve a specific purpose that is essential to your body-shaping program. As you learned earlier, you should make use of a mirror in your workout location, whether you are working out at home or elsewhere.

Mirrors allow you to see your body from different angles as you perform exercise movements. This ability to see your body as you perform the movements helps your workout in a few different ways. First and foremost, you need to know if you are performing the movement correctly to keep from injuring yourself. By checking in the mirror before, during, and after the movement, you will be able to see whether you have positioned your body correctly. Proper form is vital to increase the effectiveness of every weight-training exercise.

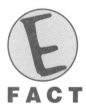

FACT

Some people split their routine so they can work every day. For example, one might work the upper body on Monday, Wednesday, and Friday; then work the lower body on Tuesday, Thursday, and Saturday. Those who split usually do the abs on both the upper- and lower-body days.

Seeing your whole body also aids in visualization—it is easier to visualize your body having the shape you are aiming for as you look at yourself performing the exercise. This total-body visualization aids in concentration and motivation. Gym mirrors are also useful to maintain a high level of "body awareness," which is conducive to a highly effective workout. The term "body awareness" as it is used in body shaping can be defined literally as the state of being aware of every part of your body at any given point in time in any given position during the exercise movement.

Mirrors in the gym also aid in increasing your "weight awareness"—that is, your awareness of where the weight is at all times in relation to where your body is. This awareness will help you to make sure the weight is lifted and caught in the correct position(s), so that the body will naturally follow suit. As you can see, floor-to-ceiling mirrors can serve to better your exercise routine. So, make sure to utilize those mirrors as you work out, because having them there is for more than just checking your hair!

Variety of Options

One more advantage to working out at a gym should be mentioned and that is that gyms are loaded with options. There's a lot more to most gyms than just free weights and weight machines. Most gyms now have large "fitness balls" by the exercise mats. So many people are now using these balls for "core" or ab work that most gyms now keep a ball or two by the mats. Balls are great for ab/core work because you have to use so many of your ab muscles to balance. Position yourself on the ball by sitting on it so that your butt and hips are resting on the ball and your back is upright, then leaning back a bit. Walk yourself forward a few steps and then back. It is a great exercise for your abs and to increase your core strength, posture, and flexibility. Of course, you can always purchase your own fitness ball and incorporate it into your home-based exercise routine. A wide variety of inexpensive fitness balls are available for purchase in the exercise sections of many stores or online.

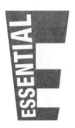

If you choose to join a gym, try to get the most for your money. If you go to the gym only once every two weeks, you're wasting both time and money. However, if you take advantage of aerobics classes and flexibility-training sessions, you're going to get a greater workout for your body as well as a greater bang for your buck.

These days, a typical gym will also offer a wide variety of aerobics classes. A selection of stationary bikes, stair climbers, treadmills, and rowing machines offer a variety of different ways to get in your aerobic workout. By working out at a gym you can perform both the weight training and the aerobic components of your program in one place. Several gyms are now offering flexibility-training sessions as well. Not to mention that after your program you can relax those sore and tired muscles in a sauna or hot tub!

Pros and Cons of Free Weights

Should you do your body-shaping workouts using free weights or machines or both? This is probably the question that is most often asked in the world of fitness. Each enthusiast and expert will have his or her own opinion based primarily on experience. The following sections will help you decide whether you should use one or the other or a combination of both. As always, allow your body to tell you what is right for you.

Pros of Free Weights

Versatile. Free weights, especially dumbbells, offer great versatility for strength training. For instance, a dumbbell exercise can be altered by holding the dumbbells with your palms facing forward, facing your body, or facing the rear. Voilà—you have three separate exercises that work your muscles in different ways. Machines, in contrast, are much more limited, with most devices allowing only one exercise apiece.

Inexpensive. Putting aside the gym membership with all its perks for a moment, you can equip your home with barbells and dumbbells for a relatively small amount of money. Of course, the more you choose to purchase, such as varying weights and accessories, the more the cost goes up. However, for the purposes of this body-shaping program, you need very little in equipment and expense to reach your goals.

Motivational lift. When working with free weights, you need to have the motivation to work the movement correctly while maintaining the desired amount of resistance. In this way, free weights allow you to better control your body's involvement and thus your mental motivation in the exercise. Whereas with machines, your body is placed in position for you and you merely perform the predetermined movement. Many people talk about the cool "feel" of the iron and the sound of the clinking metal plates of free weights as being a vital and necessary part of their workout.

Explosive action. A good many strength coaches believe that the gains derived from free weights transfer better to sports like football that require strength. What helps, they say, is that lifting heavy barbells promotes explosive bursts of power. Strength-training machines tend to control movements and to discourage explosiveness.

Muscle grouping. Some barbell exercises involve several major muscle groups at the same time. For example, lifting a barbell from the floor to the chest, then pressing it overhead utilizes the muscles from two different groups.

Similarity to natural movements. Free weights allow you to use your body in a "natural" way, simulating real-life movements accurately. You are encouraged to employ your stabilizer muscles properly and to use correct body alignment. In this way, you are using more of your body's muscles, though indirectly. For instance, when you perform a free-weight exercise standing up, you certainly target the muscles specific to that exercise, but your body must also utilize other muscles to maintain balance, just as it would in everyday life.

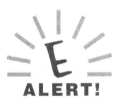

Injury can result from improper use of weights. If you remember to warm up every time before starting and if you are careful to assume the correct positioning described with each exercise, you will not hurt yourself. Correct body form is important because it forces you to place stress on the muscle being worked and not to compensate by using other areas such as the lower back, neck, and joints.

Cons of Free Weights

Safety concerns. The effectiveness of free-weight exercise depends to a great extent on using proper form. If the movements are performed incorrectly not only will you not get the benefit from the exercise, you could actually cause injury. Whereas machines will likely put your body into the proper position, you're on your own with free weights. This is why it is especially important for beginners to find a proper guideline from which to work—for instance, you can use the directions in this book or a professional instructor.

Time involved. Training with free weights can be a very time-consuming process. If you are pressed for time and want to get in a quick workout, performing a Nautilus circuit is much quicker than using free weights. When using free weights, you must ensure that your body and the weights are properly positioned and that you are performing the technique properly. This takes time to set up and execute, whereas the machines do most of this work for you. Also, in the more advanced stages of training when heavy weights are being used, some free-weight exercises require a spotter, and it may take you some time to locate a spotter for that exercise session.

Pros and Cons of Machines

While some people prefer free weights, others wouldn't even think of doing their workouts without utilizing the machines. In many ways, exercise machines are easier and more convenient to use than free weights. However, they also have their not-so-great attributes as well. If you are considering using the machines at your local gym, read through the following pros and cons to see if they would benefit your body-shaping workout.

Pros of Machines

Muscle isolation. Exercise machines are designed to target specific muscles. Because of this, they are usually safer to use in muscle isolation since it can be easy to improperly position your body when using free weights. In the same vein, when you want to experiment with new techniques or new muscle groups, using exercise machines will help you to do this in a safe manner. Machines provide you with much better control and stability and require less coordination and skill.

Time involved. Because you don't have to go around stacking plates and carrying dumbbells all the time (as with free weights), you can do an exercise session with machines in less time. With free weights, plates must be hoisted on and off the bar. With machines, there is no bending over to pick up heavy plates or dropping dumbbells on your foot. Instead, all you need to do to change the resistance of a machine is simply enter a code or insert a pin.

Directed lifting. Because machines are designed to ensure the correct movements for a lift, when you get tired you aren't going to be able to improperly use your body to compensate for the fatigue. The machine will guard against improper techniques and movements. Free weights, on the other hand, can be swung for momentum when you get tired rather than demanding the proper technique of lifting slowly and steadily.

Injury rehabilitation. Because machines isolate the specific muscles that are exercising, they are good for rehabilitating an injury or strengthening a specific body part.

Less clutter. Machines are self-contained and neat. There are no weights scattered about creating a hazard and an eyesore.

Cons of Machines

Boredom factor. One of the main disadvantages of using machines is that they do not offer you much variety and can become boring after a while. Especially if you choose to utilize the machines in a circuit, the routine can become quite monotonous and you begin to separate mind from body. As you know, it's essential that you keep your mind in tune with what your body is trying to accomplish. Using machines on a regular basis can break the mind-body connection, thus damaging your body's ability to perform at its optimum level.

One size does *not* fit all. Machines are often designed for the average-sized person and may be uncomfortable to use for a very tall or very short person or for women in particular. In general, women are smaller and have a smaller frame than men. A woman's average height is 5 feet 4 inches, while men average 5 feet 10 inches. How can one size machine fit both? It is very difficult to design a machine that will provide proper biomechanics for all individuals. This is a disadvantage that free weights do not have.

Risk of injury. Although it is generally accepted that careful instruction and training is necessary to master the art of free-weight lifting, in order to avoid injury, it is also true for the use of machines. The fact that some machines are far more complex than a dumbbell results in increased opportunity for accidents when they are used by individuals who have not been trained properly.

Applying Machines to Your Body-Shaping Program

While the body-shaping program offered in this book was designed to be done at home, you can certainly adapt it to fit the machines and equipment found in a gym. Whether you want to make use of that gym membership you already purchased, want to try something new and meet other fitness enthusiasts, or simply want to take your fitness routine up a notch, a gym may be a good choice for you. If you do choose to go to a gym and want help in transferring your body-shaping program to a program that uses gym machines, take a look at the following information. Here you will learn which machines work which body parts and thus learn how to utilize those machines in your body-shaping plan. The following exercises are described for use with common machines (both universal and nautilus are used here). Use the table on page 213 to assign the body part you want to work on to the appropriate weight machine or free-weight exercise.

Intensify Your Workout

If you're looking to make the most of your body-shaping program or to take it up a notch, you can develop a well-rounded program that will challenge the major muscle groups by adding just a few machine exercises. Adding these basic machine exercises to your body-shaping routine is a good way to experience an easy introduction to machine work and will intensify your already well-rounded workout. The following sections highlight those machine exercises that are best suited for the chest, shoulders, back, arms, legs, and calves.

Body Part	Machine	Comparable Free-Weight Exercise
Chest	Pec Dec, bench press machine	Dumbbell Chest Flyes and Forearm Touches, Dumbbell Presses on a Bench or Mat
Shoulders	Nautilus double shoulder machine, Nautilus deltoid machine	Lateral Raises with Dumbbells, Shoulder Press with Dumbbells
Arms	Nautilus biceps machine, Universal triceps press-down	Standing Alternate Biceps Curls with Dumbbells, Seated Two-Arm Triceps Extensions
Legs	Leg-press machine, Nautilus leg-extension machine	Squats with Unweighted Bar, Lunges with Unweighted Bar, and/or Leg Extensions with Ankle Weights, Leg Curls with Ankle Weights
Hips and thighs	Hip and thigh abductor and adductor machine	Inner-thigh Lifts and Side Leg Raises
Abs	Ab crunch machine	Classic and Oblique Crunches
Back	Lat pull-down machine, cable rows	Bent-Over Rowing with Unweighted Bar, Good Mornings
Buttocks	Back leg tucks with cables	Buttock Tighteners, Rear Leg Scissors
Calf	Seated calf press	Standing Toe Raises

Bench Press

The bench press machine works the chest (pectoral) and rear arm (triceps) muscles, with help from the shoulder (anterior deltoid) muscles. To use this machine, lie face-up on the bench with your buttocks, shoulders, and head firmly pressed down. Keep your feet flat on the floor. Grip the bar with palms facing away from you and about shoulder-width apart. Push the bar to arm's length, pause at the top of the movement, then lower slowly and repeat.

Overhead Military Press

This exercise works the shoulder (deltoid) and triceps muscles. To use this machine, sit up with your back straight. If needed, you can use an upright bench to support your back. Grab the bar in front of you with your palms facing away from your body and hands shoulder-width apart, and keep your elbows out to the sides. Press the bar to arm's length, pause at the top of the movement, then lower slowly and repeat.

Row

This exercise works the large upper-back muscles (latissimi dorsi, or "lats"). To use this machine, sit straight with your chest against the chest pad, which can be adjusted. Grasp the handles with a thumbs-up grip. Raise the weights while concentrating on pulling with your upper-back muscles rather than your biceps, which will assist a bit. Lower slowly and repeat.

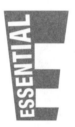

While the exercises listed here will give your body a great workout, you can also add exercises for the hamstrings, abdominals, back extensors, neck, and forearms as the next step toward a total body program.

Biceps Curl

This exercise works the front arm muscles (biceps). To use this machine, sit up straight with your chest against the chest pad. Your arms should be completely extended and resting on top of the bench with your elbows positioned lower than your shoulders. Grab the bar with your palms up and hands slightly less than shoulder-width apart. Curl the bar up to your chin, pause at the top of the movement, then lower slowly and repeat. To avoid elbow stress, don't lock your elbows, and be sure to keep your biceps tensed when the arms are extending.

Leg Press

This exercise works the large thigh (quadriceps) muscles and hip extensors (gluteus maximus and hamstrings). When using this machine, your legs should be extended completely; you can adjust the chair to fit you. Sit up straight and keep your lower back and buttocks firmly pressed against the chair. Your knees should be bent to a 90-degree angle with your feet flat on the pedals. Holding onto the chair's handles, push the pedals until your knees are straight. Be sure to keep your knees unlocked. Hold this position as you concentrate on the muscles being used, then lower slowly and repeat.

Calf Raise

This exercise works the lower-leg muscles (gastrocnemius and soleus). This is a seated exercise because sitting isolates the calves better and promotes better form. Adjust the seat to allow a 90-degree knee bend with the resistance pad slightly above your knees. Allow for complete ankle motion. Place your toes and the ball of each foot on the foot pad. Pushing with your calves, raise your knees as high as possible (this also raises the stack of weights). Hold the position for a moment as you feel the muscles tense, then lower slowly and repeat.

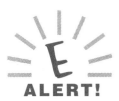

ALERT!

Always be sure you know how to use a machine before you use it. If you don't know how, ask someone. To try to go it alone could cause you serious injury. It's better to be safe than sorry.

Gym Etiquette

Some people view the gym as a subculture all unto itself. While this may sound a little suspect, it's really not all too far off. There is a class structure that is divided based upon physical fitness, a language that only the members understand and speak, and a set of unspoken rules that should be followed lest you be frowned upon. That said, not everyone takes his or her gym experiences so seriously. In fact, those who go there to tone their bodies *and* have fun are the people who give the gym its flavorful atmosphere. Even so, these people know and follow (for the most part) the rules of gym etiquette.

As you walk into the gym, take a look around and see if there are rules posted throughout the building. Sometimes you will see rules asking you to wipe down the machines you use, return weights to their appropriate places on the racks, and to only spend a certain amount of time on the cardio equipment. This is all well and good, and you should certainly pay attention to these rather obvious rules, but what about those rules of etiquette that aren't written down for everyone to see?

Don't Be Pushy

If you are at a gym and someone is using the machine you want to use, you should politely stand off to the side until she is done. Do not crowd the person or break her concentration by hovering or trying to rush her through her movement. When she steps away, ask if she is finished in case she is just taking a rest interval between sets. If she is taking a rest interval between sets, you may ask if you can "work in" with her, which means that you alternate sets with her on the same machine— you work while she rests and vice versa.

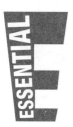

> If you see someone headed for the machine you were just thinking of using, don't race ahead of the person and smugly grin when you've won the race. Cutting in line wasn't acceptable in elementary school and it's not acceptable in the gym.

The gym is not a bar; hence, it is not a place to practice your latest and greatest pickup line. Trying to strike up a conversation with someone who is having a hard enough time catching her breath on the treadmill isn't going to get you very far. Most people go to the gym to work out, not to try to find dates or make new friends. If you are persistent in your conversational tactics, you are likely being too pushy. Back off, get your workout done, and then go to the bar.

Keep Your Workspace Clean

Most gyms keep paper towels and spray bottles near all the machines. If not, always bring a towel with you. You are supposed to spray and wipe down any surfaces your body touched when you used the machine. Don't do a half-hearted swipe! Give the surface a good wipe to get rid of your sweat! You wouldn't want to sit in a pool of sweat left by someone else, so pay the same courtesy to those who will follow you.

You should also pick up and return any weights used to their proper locations. This is common courtesy. The left-out weights could be in the way of the next person wanting to use that bench or area for his or her workout or could easily cause someone to trip and fall.

Don't Stare

It's never polite to stare and at the gym is no exception. Granted it may be very tempting to goggle at the scantily clad gods and goddesses strutting their stuff, but it's not a good idea for more reasons than one. First of all, by staring at others you are breaking your concentration. It's been stressed throughout this book that you need the proper focus and concentration to make the most of each workout session. If you are watching someone else, you aren't paying attention to what you're doing, and at best this could slow your efforts and at worst you could hurt yourself.

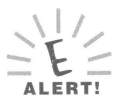

ALERT!

The mirrors are there so you can check your form and make sure you are performing an exercise correctly. They are not there so that you can fix your hair, apply makeup, or model your latest workout wear.

Another reason you shouldn't stare is simply because it's rude. Think of how you feel when someone is staring at you. Now place yourself in a situation (such as a gym) in which many people are self-conscious enough about their bodies, and the staring just adds undue stress. Granted, there are some who go to the gym so they *will* be stared at, but for the most part, others are there to get their business done and leave. Even the best-looking people can be made to feel uncomfortable with staring. Pay everyone else the same courtesy you would expect from them.

Miscellaneous Rules of Etiquette

A little common sense and a lot of common courtesy will make your visit to the gym much more pleasurable. Just in case you are slightly lacking in either of those areas, take a look at some of the following rules of gym etiquette.

- Don't criticize others.
- Don't throw weights around.
- Don't chat on your cell phone while trying to work out.
- Always clean up after yourself: This includes in the bathroom.
- Do give others their personal space.
- Don't monopolize equipment or space.
- Keep noises to a minimum. This includes music, grunts, and temper tantrums.
- Wear appropriate clothing.
- Don't bring food into the gym.
- Don't try to compete with those around you.

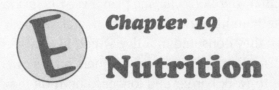

Chapter 19

Nutrition

Body shaping is a program that advocates a combination of targeted exercise supplemented by aerobic activity for weight loss and a sensible eating plan. The only way to achieve long-lasting changes to your body is to maintain the body-shaping lifestyle over time. This calls for an awareness of sound nutritional principles and the development of healthy eating habits.

Why Bother with Nutrition?

Many people work under the assumption that if they are exercising, they can eat whatever they want. While some people are able to eat hoards of fatty foods and not seem to gain an ounce, this is only harming their bodies in the long run. In order to be healthy and fit, you must incorporate a sensible eating plan within your body-shaping plan. Everyone's body functions differently. Some have high metabolic rates that allow them to burn off whatever calories they consume in a day, which in turn keeps their weight stable or causes them to lose weight. Others have slower metabolic rates and have to work harder and longer to burn off the calories they consume. Regardless of your metabolic rate, you need to watch what you eat if you want to be healthy and have the energy needed to maintain your body-shaping regimen.

Maintaining Your Body Shape

Another factor to consider when evaluating the value of eating right is how diet can help you keep the body you have worked so hard for. Once you put so much effort into improving your appearance, you want to do what you can to maintain the developed muscles that have toned and tightened your body. Serious bodybuilders know the importance of a good diet and any review of bodybuilding literature will reveal that a good percentage of it is devoted to nutrition and diet. A bodybuilder's goal is different from yours but the methods will be the same. While a bodybuilder's ultimate nutritional goal is to reduce the amount of body fat to its absolute minimum in order to help show off their massive muscle bulk, one of your nutritional goals will be to nourish the muscles you have built so they maintain their size and quality.

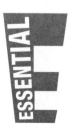

Bodybuilders also eat the foods that will fuel their energy level for their intense workouts. In addition, a major focus of their food selection is to choose foods that will build muscle. Again, while you are on a body-shaping plan, not a bodybuilding one, many of the nutritional goals will be the same, just on a much more modified level of intensity.

Nutritional Programs

Before you can begin to follow a nutritional program you must first find out what and how much you need to eat in order to have enough energy to perform and sustain your workouts, get to and maintain your desired weight, and help your new muscles grow and stay nourished. There are as many "food plans" and diets out there as there are people to follow them. You may have tried a few yourself. This book will not advocate one or two over and above the rest—that task is way beyond the scope of this chapter. Instead, you will learn a few sound nutritional principles that fit in with your body-shaping program. You will have enough basic information to formulate your own personalized eating plan. The next chapter will provide sample recipes for foods that are indicated for those who are following a fitness program such as this one, while this chapter will provide enough information for you to understand why those foods are suggested.

Well-Known Diets

If you already have a food program that works for you, by all means stick with it. If it is working for you, chances are it is based on sound nutritional principles, unless of course you are on some fad diet like the watermelon diet, the popcorn diet, or the ice cream diet! Opinions vary and even medical experts disagree on which one of the well-known diets such as the Zone, Atkins, Pritikin, and others is the one to follow.

These issues cannot be resolved here, so suffice it to say that controversial food programs will be avoided and only the most widely accepted nutritional concepts will be presented for your use in this program.

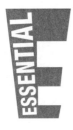

A good rule of thumb is that moderation and balance are always wise. You need to enjoy a variety of foods, not too much or too little of any one food, and stay away from high-fat, high-calorie foods in general. Stick to the basics—include more fruits, vegetables, fiber, and sources of quality protein, and reduce your intake of fat and refined sugar.

USDA Food Guide Pyramid

A valuable guide in choosing your foods would be to bear in mind the principles set forth in the USDA Food Guide Pyramid. The Food Guide Pyramid is a research-based food guidance system developed by the U.S. Department of Agriculture and supported by the Department of Health and Human Services.

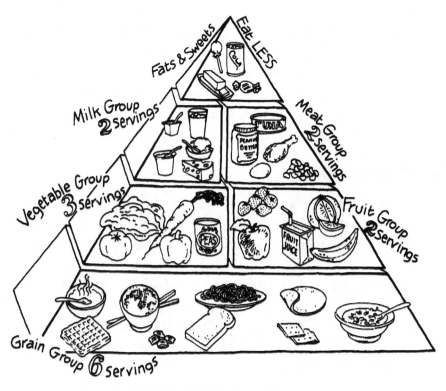

▲ USDA Food Guide Pyramid

The pyramid separates food into five major groups and recommends a certain number of servings from each of the five groups for good overall nutritional health. The five groups are as follows:

1. Milk, yogurt, and cheese
2. Meat, poultry, fish, dry beans, eggs, and nuts
3. Vegetables

4. Fruits
5. Bread, cereal, rice, and pasta

In addition to defining the five major food groups, and recommending a certain number of servings from each, the pyramid goes on to set forth some general dietary guidelines. The government's seven dietary guidelines are as follows:

1. Eat a variety of foods.
2. Balance the food you eat with physical activity—maintain or improve your weight.
3. Choose a diet with plenty of grain products, vegetables, and fruits.
4. Choose a diet low in fat, saturated fat, and cholesterol.
5. Choose a diet moderate in sugars.
6. Choose a diet moderate in salt and sodium.
7. If you drink alcoholic beverages, do it in moderation.

The USDA Food Guide Pyramid was developed in such a way that if its serving guidelines are followed, one would get the right proportion of the U.S. Recommended Dietary Allowances (RDAs) for protein, minerals, vitamins, and dietary fiber. Moreover, following the serving guidelines will ensure a reduction or even elimination of such harmful dietary practices as eating excess calories, fat, saturated fat, cholesterol, sodium, and sugars.

Although the USDA Food Guide Pyramid has its detractors, and many of the more popular food programs and diets embrace principles that are contradictory to the principles set forth in the pyramid, generally it is considered to be a high-quality tool to improve one's diet. The emphasis on variety and portion control helps ensure the consumption of a balance of good food and its high-fiber/low-fat guideline is a sound nutritional principle.

Your Personal Food Plan

Depending on your own personal needs, likes and dislikes, and the amount of weight you need to lose, you can construct your own food plan using the principles of good nutrition as a starting point. Before you can start, let's make sure you have a good grasp of the nutritional value of the food you like to eat.

The following sections will provide a quick review of some terms that are used frequently in dietary discussions, and an understanding of them is essential to develop a plan for yourself that is sensible and well balanced.

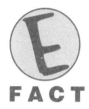

FACT

Cellulite is a concern for many women. Cellulite is a deposit of fat that creates a dimpled look. As you know, the best way to get rid of fat is to add an aerobic portion to your body-shaping regimen and eat sensibly.

Protein

There is more controversy surrounding the quantity of protein that is good for you than practically any other food issue. While no expert disputes the importance of protein to the diet, there is major disagreement about how much is good for you and how much is too much. Because excess protein that is not used by the body is stored as body fat, unlimited consumption of protein may not be advisable. As in most things, balance is the key—too little protein and your body may not function properly and too much and the excess will be stored as fat. Critics of the high-protein diet also warn against unlimited consumption because so many protein sources are high in saturated fat.

The importance of protein to a fitness lifestyle cannot be underestimated. Protein is the building block of muscle tissue. Protein supplies the body with amino acids. Protein functions to maintain and repair muscle and other tissues; make hemoglobin, which carries oxygen to exercising muscles; form antibodies to fight infection and disease; and produce enzymes and hormones that regulate body processes. If carbohydrates and fats are not consumed in sufficient quantities to meet the body's energy needs, then the body will turn to protein as a last resort.

Good sources of protein include:

- Milk and yogurt
- Lean red meat such as top round and sirloin steak
- Legumes such as beans and peas
- Chicken and turkey breast
- Eggs
- Cottage cheese
- Lobster, salmon, shrimp, crab, and haddock
- Nuts
- Soy (the only complete vegetable protein)

Carbohydrates

Carbohydrates are important to the body-shaping lifestyle because they are the body's main source of energy. Carbohydrates are particularly important if your fitness program is based in large part on weight-training activity because they are the only source of glycogen, which is a substance critical to muscle health.

In the body, carbohydrates from foods are converted into blood sugar, or glucose. Whatever is not burned up immediately for energy is stored in the body as glycogen. When you exercise, your muscles draw on the glycogen for energy. Since it is not stored in great quantities, the body needs a steady stream of carbohydrates coming in to replace it. This is why athletes and fitness enthusiasts consider carbohydrates to be the most important nutrient.

Two Categories

Carbohydrates are broken up into two categories: complex carbohydrates and simple carbohydrates. Complex carbohydrates usually consist of starches and dietary fiber. Some examples of complex carbohydrates are potatoes, rice, pasta, some vegetables, bread, and cereal. Complex carbohydrates tend to be low in calories and fat, and high in fiber. Because the breaking down of complex carbohydrates is a gradual process that takes some time, your blood sugar and energy level will remain fairly stable during the breakdown process.

Simple carbohydrates are simply sugar! Not just the kind you find in the sugar bowl on the table, but also the kind that is found in milk and fruit, for example. Simple carbohydrates are absorbed quickly and cause great fluctuations in the blood sugar levels. Think about the "sugar highs" kids get at birthday parties when they eat all that ice cream and candy and soda, and then spend the next hour climbing the walls and swinging from the chandeliers. This is true with adults as well, even though the symptoms are not as obvious! Sugar-heavy foods do more damage than just creating mood highs and lows, and a good general rule of thumb is to avoid them because they are mostly high in "empty" calories and supply no nutritional value.

Acceptable sugar substitutes are Splenda, an artificial sweetener that can even be used in baking, and Stevia, a natural sweetener that comes from the leaves of a plant found in South America. Both of these calorie-free sugar substitutes do not affect insulin levels, so they do not cause the highs and lows that sugar does.

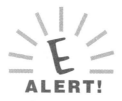

ALERT!

Be wary of labels: Sugar is hidden in many foods. Although a food label may not list sugar, you should check carefully for the following words, which signal sugar. If they are first, second, or third on the list of ingredients, you should leave the item on the shelf: high fructose corn syrup, dextrose, fructose, fruit juice concentrate, glucose, honey, lactose, maltose, molasses, sucrose, and syrup.

A Word about Fiber

During digestion, all carbohydrates except fiber break down into sugar. Some fiber is soluble, that is, it can break down later in the intestines. This happens with the fiber found in oats, beans, and soy-based foods. Soluble fiber is good for those who are trying to lower their cholesterol. Other types of fiber such as wheat bran are insoluble, that is, they pass right through the digestive tract and out. Fiber is found only in plant foods and is an important part of any diet. It can help you feel fuller sooner so you eat less, and it has been linked with lower rates of heart disease, colon cancer, and diabetes.

Sources of Carbohydrates

Good sources of quality carbohydrates are:

- Whole-grain breads
- Pasta
- Oatmeal
- High-fiber cereals such as wheat bran
- Potatoes and sweet potatoes
- Steamed brown and wild rice
- Barley, beans, and corn
- Squash, pumpkins, and yams
- Strawberries, apples, melons, and oranges

Fat

In spite of what most people believe, not all fats are "bad" fats. Certain amounts of fat are essential for important bodily tasks such as the absorption of particular vitamins and for proper hormonal functioning. Essentially, fats are concentrated fuel. Primary sources of fat are animal foods such as meat, poultry, and dairy products. Saturated fats are solid at room temperature and are the fats that have cholesterol and contribute to the clogging of the arteries and increase your risk for heart disease. Unsaturated fats are better for your health and are usually found in fish and vegetables.

Fats are generally dense in calories and provide twice as much energy as carbohydrates and protein. However, be careful because although fats can be the best source of energy, the excess calories found in them can lead to unwanted weight gain. Fats also supply essential fatty acids.

Although you obviously need fat in your diet, it is important that you choose your fats wisely. You should cut back your intake of saturated fats. Some examples of saturated fats are butter, lard, and tropical vegetable oils such as palm and coconut. A good rule of thumb is that if it is solid at room temperature (butter, margarine, and shortening), it should be avoided. Hydrogenated fats and trans fats (check your labels) should also be avoided.

Examples of good fats are oils such as safflower, sesame, canola, and olive oil. Another example of a good fat is the fat found in an avocado. Overall, though, fats should be kept to a minimum for good health. The American Heart Association recommends that not more than 30 percent of our daily calorie intake come from fat, and saturated fats should not be more than 10 percent of that amount.

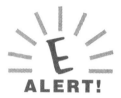

ALERT!

Beware of labels. Lately there has been a flood of new products on the shelves boasting various versions of the "low," "reduced," or "nonfat" claim. Be very wary of these products because the labeling criteria is misleading at best and some foods that claim to be reduced fat might not be as low in fat as you think. Also, it is good to remember that these foods are generally very high in calories.

Vitamins

Vitamins assist in the growth of body tissues and help the body release energy for fuel. Vitamin deficiencies can affect physical performance, since vitamins regulate carbohydrate, protein, and fat metabolism.

As stated before, a diet that follows the USDA Food Pyramid should provide you with your recommended daily quantity of vitamins and minerals. However, the vitamin supplement business is a multibillion-dollar industry for a reason, and many people swear by the benefits they say they receive from taking extra vitamins. Some people even take at least ten times the RDA (Recommended Dietary Allowance) on a daily basis.

Megadosing with vitamins can be very harmful to your health and is not recommended by most experts. Some vitamin supplements taken to excess can cause damage to the body. For example, fat-soluble vitamins such as A and D can be stored in your body and produce toxic symptoms. Even water-soluble vitamins such as niacin and B_6 can cause adverse effects when taken in large doses. Sometimes they can block the good effect of other vitamins that you need. Vitamin C taken to excess can cause gastrointestinal distress and diarrhea. Large doses of iron can not only cause iron toxicity, but also block the proper absorption of magnesium and zinc. Often, people who take massive doses of certain vitamins do not realize that the body can only metabolize a certain amount at a time and most of the dose is excreted through the urine anyway. At the current sticker price of vitamin supplements, that is some expensive urine!

If you are embarking on your body-shaping program and want to be sure your body has enough energy to sustain your efforts, your best bet is to make sure you follow a healthy food program. Taking extra vitamins is not a good substitute for a proper meal plan.

Food high in vitamins should be a large part of your food plan. For example, foods high in vitamins E, A, and C are:

- Carrots
- Milk and skim milk
- Peanuts
- Orange juice
- Broccoli
- Spinach
- Strawberries

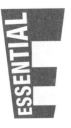

If you eat a well-balanced variety of nutritious foods, using the Food Pyramid as your guide for determining your daily intake, you should be able to create a sensible eating plan that will complement your body-shaping efforts.

Water

Whether you are following a body-shaping plan or not, it is important to drink adequate amounts of fluids, especially water, every day. Water is an essential nutrient for life and health, second only to oxygen in importance to your body. You can live longer without food than you can without water! You should drink at least eight to ten large glasses of water daily. If you are on a regular exercise program, which you should be if you are reading this book, you will require even more water than the minimum just described. Figure on adding at least an additional glass of water for each fifteen minutes that you work out. So, if your workout lasts an hour, that is four extra glasses of water a day.

At first, it might take some extra effort to ensure that you meet these water intake requirements, but after a while you will become accustomed to drinking so much water that your body will crave it when you don't have it. Get in the habit of carrying a water bottle wherever you go. Keep one in your office, your bag, your bedroom, your kitchen, everywhere you spend time. Purchase one of those nylon water bottle holders that keep the water cold and have a shoulder strap for ease of carrying. Save your empty bottles and fill them three-quarters full with water and stick them in the freezer. Before you go out, open it and fill it the rest of the way with your water (whatever your source may be—some buy water in large bottles or filter it with a home device, while, for some, tap water is fine). Take it with you wherever you are going and it will stay cold for a long time. Create some other tips and tricks of your own to help you remember to drink your daily requirement of water. (E)

Chapter 20

E Sample Body-Shaping Recipes

This chapter does not pretend to present a comprehensive eating plan. Instead, it will offer a collection of recipes for healthy, sensible meals, ideas for quick, nutritious snacks, and a sampling of delicious high-protein and low-fat smoothies, all meant to complement your body-shaping exercise plan.

Smoothies

For nutritional value, ease of preparation, and good taste, too, smoothies are a great choice! Smoothies are popular with people trying to lose weight because they offer a quick way to obtain important vitamins and other essential nutrients in a simple, easy-to-prepare shake. Also, smoothies are a popular way to boost your protein intake. For those of you who do not particularly like to eat too much meat, protein drinks are a lifesaver since protein is so important to the body shaper and bodybuilder who is attempting to build muscle. If you are developing muscle, you need good quantities of lean, high-quality protein that contains the seven essential amino acids (there are nine total essential amino acids) for muscle growth and repair, and smoothies can deliver that.

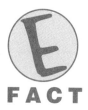

FACT

These recipes are nutritious and follow the general guidelines for healthy eating. Some of them will be examples of low-fat recipes, others will be examples of high-protein, low-carb recipes, and some will be examples of recipes that provide important quantities of fresh vegetables and fiber, but all will be examples of good, wholesome, nutritious foods.

Making Smoothies

You can make smoothies in a blender, or special "smoothie machines" are available now for die-hard smoothie pros. If you do not have a blender, do not despair! Most protein powders and shake mixes for sale advertise the fact that their powder is easily blendable, and you just need to shake the container well by hand for a smooth shake.

A few recipes are included in this section, but basically the idea of a smoothie is to use a powder as a base (if you desire), put in your chosen liquid (usually either water, milk, or juice), add some ice cubes, and mix in your chosen solid ingredients, such as strawberries, blueberries, bananas, and/or yogurt.

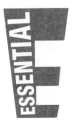

As you begin to create your own smoothies, you will likely come across a few tips and special ingredients. But to get you started, here's a secret smoothie-making tip: Freeze your fruit juice before using it in a smoothie. This makes your drink frostier.

Smoothie Products

Most fitness enthusiasts buy special powders and premixed drinks in health food stores and supermarkets, but this is not necessary. If you do choose to use them, though, read labels carefully because there are important differences among the many shake formulas available, and depending on what your particular nutritional objective is, you might end up purchasing an expensive powder that will do the opposite of what you desire.

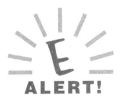

Because there are so many differing opinions as to which diet or food plan is the "one" to follow, no one diet is recommended here. Instead, this is a collection of various nutritious recipes that you can use and adapt to your own personal chosen food plan.

No matter what your diet goal is, whether it is to lose weight or gain weight, whether you are on a low-fat or low-carb diet plan, the first suggestion is that you avoid the meal-replacement shakes and powders that are so heavily advertised. These shakes make lots of diet promises, but if you study the ingredient list you will discover that an 8-ounce serving can be loaded with sugars such as sucrose, fructose, dextrose, artificial flavors, and that they can pack as much as 250 calories, 9 grams of fat, and 45 grams of carbs! Many contain ephedra (ma huang), which is a stimulant and considered by many to be dangerous to take. Though they do have essential vitamins and minerals, what they provide can easily be obtained by taking one multivitamin.

It is strongly recommended that if you are going to buy powders as a base for your smoothies, you stick to the ones that have a protein base (usually whey) and use Splenda or sucralose as a sweetener, instead of dextrose, fructose, and sucrose. Check your calorie, fat, and carb counts. Even if you are on a low-fat diet and not counting carbs, why buy one with 45 grams of carbs when you can get one with the same ingredients and only 12 or 4 grams of carbs? Most shake mixes should not have more than 200 calories or 4 grams of fat per serving.

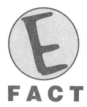

FACT

If you find a brand you like, stick with it. Most come in a variety of flavors, not only vanilla, chocolate, and strawberry, but also orange-banana crème, and a host of other creative flavor blends. Have fun with them!

High-Protein Smoothie
Serves 1

This is a basic protein mix for someone on a low-carb diet. The other smoothies in this recipe section all have fruit and should be avoided by low-carbers because of the high carb content of fruit. Instead, use the recipe here and vary it by adding other "safe" low-carb ingredients. Be creative and have fun inventing variations to this basic protein shake.

1 cup water
2 scoops vanilla-flavored whey protein powder
1 packet or 1 teaspoon Splenda, if the powder is not already sweetened
2 tablespoons heavy whipping cream
¼ teaspoon vanilla extract
Dash of cinnamon
6 ice cubes

Combine all ingredients in a blender, adding the ice last. Mix until well blended and frothy.

◆ ◆ ◆

Basic Low-Fat, High-Protein Fruit Smoothie

Serves 1

Here is a colorful fruit smoothie for those who are on a low-fat plan. Remember, you still need the protein! If you prefer soy milk, feel free to use that instead of the regular milk.

1 cup skim or low-fat milk
2 scoops protein powder
1 packet or 1 teaspoon Splenda, if protein powder is not sweetened or sweet enough
½ banana
4–5 strawberries (you can also use frozen strawberries)
1 cup nonfat yogurt, vanilla or plain
Dash of cinnamon or drop of honey
¼ teaspoon vanilla extract (optional)
6 ice cubes

Combine all ingredients in the blender, adding the ice cubes last. Blend until smooth and frothy.

◆ ◆ ◆

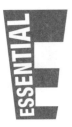

If you want to kick it up a notch, put a tablespoon full of wheat germ or bran in your smoothies. This will provide a drink that is full of B vitamins. Or, for a jolt of calcium, stir in a tablespoon of nonfat dry instant milk powder while blending. One tablespoon provides 60 milligrams of calcium.

Blue Skies Energizer

Serves 1

The blue color may be calming, but the effect is energizing!

$^2/_3$ cup fresh or frozen blueberries
1 cup skim or low-fat milk
2 egg whites (optional)
$^1/_2$ teaspoon vanilla extract
1 packet or 1 teaspoon Splenda
6 ice cubes

Combine all ingredients in a blender, adding the ice cubes last. Mix until smooth and frothy.

Strawberry-Banana Crush

Serves 1

You can use fresh or frozen strawberries—but if you use frozen, be sure to buy the unsweetened kind.

1 cup apple juice
1 ripe banana
6 fresh or frozen strawberries
2 egg whites (optional)
1 packet or 1 teaspoon Splenda
$^1/_2$ cup vanilla or plain yogurt
6 ice cubes

Combine all ingredients in blender, adding the ice last. Blend until well mixed and smooth and frothy.

Wraps

When you want to imply how fabulous something is, the saying goes like this: "It's the best invention since sliced bread." Well, ever since wraps arrived on the food scene, we suspect that saying will be changed to say "the best invention since wraps!" Wraps have become enormously popular with anyone wanting to cut down on the intake of bread but still enjoy the versatility and convenience of a sandwich. Wraps come in all flavors from plain and whole wheat to spinach and tomato, garlic, sun-dried tomato, and cheese. They can be found at any supermarket these days. For the low-carb eater, there are even low-carb wraps available online from any of the special low-carb Web sites listed in the resources section at the back of the book.

Wraps can be used in a variety of ways. Feel free to experiment and enjoy the varieties of wraps. They can be used with meat and cheese sandwich fillings, veggie fillings, or even with cheese for a quick quesadilla.

Cheese and Chicken Quesadilla

Serves 1 for a meal or 2 for a snack

This version of the famous Mexican quick "sandwich" is adapted here for a quick nutritious snack or lunch.

Nonstick cooking spray
2 soft wraps, any flavor
½ cup grated Cheddar cheese
½ cup cooked shredded chicken
¼ cup salsa

1. Spray a flat griddle or grill with cooking spray. After it heats up, place both wraps flat on the grill, spread the cheese and chicken on the top of each wrap, and let it heat through. After a few minutes, fold each wrap in half. Press down on the tops with your spatula. Flip the wraps and cook on the other side for about 2 more minutes, until all the cheese inside is melted.
2. Remove to a platter and cut the folded wraps in half. You should have 4 quarters. Serve with salsa.

◆ ◆ ◆

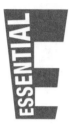

Try these fillings for wraps: Ham and cheese; bacon, lettuce, and tomato; turkey and cheese; cream cheese and ham; scrambled eggs with peppers and onions; tuna salad; peanut butter and jelly; or just use your imagination!

Chicken Fajitas

Serves 4

Quick and easy to prepare, this low-fat dish is great fun to cook and eat.

2 pounds boneless, skinless chicken breasts
¼ cup lime juice
¼ cup olive oil
1 clove garlic, minced
½ teaspoon ground cumin
1 yellow onion, peeled and sliced
1 green bell pepper, cored and sliced
Nonstick cooking spray
4 wraps or tortillas
Salsa
Sour cream
Guacamole

1. Cut the chicken into 2-inch strips and place them in a glass bowl with the lime juice, olive oil, garlic, and cumin. Marinate for 15 to 20 minutes and then add the onion and pepper slices. Stir to mix well with the marinade.

2. After the vegetables and chicken have marinated for another 15 minutes, drain the marinade and heat a grill or griddle. Spray the grill with nonstick cooking spray, then place the chicken, onion, and peppers on the hot grill. The grill should be so hot that the peppers, onions, and chicken sizzle and cook rapidly.

3. When the chicken is cooked through (white in color, no longer pink inside), remove the meat and veggies from the grill and serve immediately with warmed wraps or tortillas, salsa, sour cream, and guacamole.

Quick Meals, Lunches, and Dinners

Finding time to fit your workout into your daily busy schedule is difficult; finding time to plan and prepare wholesome, nutritious meals that support your workout is yet another challenge. With some careful menu planning and some thought to planning out a few days of meals in advance, you can successfully maintain the progress you are making with your body-shaping program. One great idea is to prepare foods that can be made ahead of time, refrigerated, taken with you to the office or gym, eaten while on the move, and prepared quickly when arriving home after a full day of work. This section contains some suggestions for wholesome, nutritious foods that fit these criteria.

Another reason to try the foods in this section is that they fit the bill for those who subscribe to the theory that several small meals eaten throughout the day is better for weight loss. Known as "grazing," this diet theory maintains that by eating several smaller meals throughout the day, you keep your metabolism revved, your blood sugar levels stable, and your hunger at bay.

Portobello Burgers

Serves 2

Portobello mushrooms are the vegetarian's answer to the hamburger. They are meaty and tasty and can be grilled and eaten on a sandwich roll, too.

2 portobello mushrooms	2 slices mozzarella or Swiss cheese
1 tablespoon olive oil	Salt and pepper, to taste

1. Remove and discard the stems from the mushroom caps and wipe the caps clean with a damp paper towel. Brush the mushrooms with olive oil. Heat a grill or nonstick skillet and cook the portobellos for 3 to 4 minutes on each side. After turning them once, put 1 slice of the cheese on the top of the cooked side of each mushroom.

2. When the cheese melts, remove the mushrooms from the frying pan and place on a dish. Sprinkle with salt and pepper. Serve on a whole-wheat roll with lettuce and tomato, if desired.

◆ ◆ ◆

Bowl of Red

Serves 6

Fix this zesty chili on the weekend and make enough to pack a bowl for a quick, microwaveable lunch for the next few days.

1½ pounds beef sirloin, cubed
1 tablespoon olive oil
1 yellow cooking onion, peeled and diced
2 cloves garlic, peeled and minced
2 tablespoons chili powder
1 teaspoon dried oregano
1 tablespoon ground cumin
1 tablespoon sweet paprika
1 tablespoon unsweetened cocoa powder
1 tablespoon instant coffee granules
1 teaspoon salt
2 cups water
1 (12- or 16-ounce) can diced tomatoes
1 can kidney beans, drained
1 medium white onion, diced (for topping)
2 cups grated Cheddar cheese (for topping)
2 cups sour cream (for topping)

1. Brown the meat in a nonstick skillet until it loses its pink color and is cooked throughout. Remove the meat to a bowl and drain off the fat.
2. Add the olive oil and chopped onion to the same skillet and sauté the onion. When the onion is soft and transparent, add the garlic, chili powder, oregano, cumin, paprika, cocoa powder, instant coffee, and salt; stir well. Add the water and bring to a low simmer, stirring gently throughout to blend. Immediately add the tomatoes and return the meat to the pan. Simmer on low for 1 hour.
3. Ten minutes before serving, stir in the beans and heat throughout. You can also serve with sour cream, chopped fresh onion, and grated Cheddar cheese.

Mozzarella and Tomato Salad

Serves 1 as a meal or 2 as a side

What a simple but wonderful dish to have when the basil is fresh and the tomatoes are ripe! Try to find fresh basil—it tastes so much better than dried basil.

  4 large ripe tomatoes
  Salt and pepper, to taste
  ½ pound fresh mozzarella cheese
  1 bunch fresh basil
  ¼ cup virgin olive oil

1. Wash the tomatoes and pat them dry. Slice the tomatoes and arrange the slices in a slightly overlapping row across the middle of a serving dish. Sprinkle lightly with salt and pepper.

2. Gently put a thin slice of mozzarella cheese on top of each slice of tomato, keeping the overlapping pattern. Lightly chop a handful of fresh basil leaves into large shreds and sprinkle over the tomatoes and cheese. Drizzle the olive oil over the top and serve.

London Broil with Asian Marinade
Serves 6–8

Serve with a large mixed green salad for a complete meal. The next day, the leftover slices are great in a wrap for a sandwich.

- $1/3$ cup low-salt (sodium) soy sauce
- 2 tablespoons dry sherry
- 1 tablespoon sesame oil
- 1 tablespoon rice vinegar
- 1 garlic clove, minced
- 1 tablespoon honey
- 1 teaspoon fresh-grated ginger
- 3-pound London broil

1. Mix together all the ingredients except the meat in a large nonreactive baking dish. Pierce the meat all over with a fork (this allows the marinade to seep in) and place it in the marinade. Let marinate for 2 to 3 hours or overnight in the refrigerator, turning the meat a few times while it marinates.

2. Preheat a grill or the broiler and cook the meat for at least 5 to 8 minutes on each side for medium-rare, basting during the cooking. When the steak is done, slice it against the grain on a diagonal.

Greek Chicken Thighs

Serves 4

These flavorful thighs are tender from marinating in the lemon juice, and they taste great, too! Serve with a mixed green or Greek salad (see recipe following).

> ¼ cup olive oil
> Juice from 1 lemon
> 2 tablespoons dried oregano
> 3 cloves garlic, peeled and minced
> Salt and pepper, to taste
> 6 boneless, skinless chicken thighs

1. In a glass bowl, mix together the olive oil, lemon juice, oregano, garlic, salt, and pepper. Wash and dry the chicken, then place it in the marinade. Cover and let marinate in the refrigerator for at least 3 hours or overnight.

2. Preheat the broiler. Drain off and discard the marinade, and place the chicken in a broiling pan. Broil for 5 to 10 minutes on each side. To be sure the chicken is cooked, pierce it with a fork and make sure the juice runs clear or slice into a corner of one of the pieces.

Greek Salad

Serves 1 as a main dish or 2 as a side dish

This classic salad is a favorite of dieters, especially when ordering at restaurants. The feta is practically a guilt-free cheese because of its low fat content.

1 head romaine lettuce
4 cherry tomatoes
½ cucumber, peeled and sliced
½ green bell pepper, cored and sliced
¼ red onion, thinly sliced
4–6 black olives
¼ pound feta cheese, crumbled

For the dressing, blend together:

¼ cup olive oil
⅛ cup balsamic vinegar
½ teaspoon crumbled oregano
Salt and pepper to taste
½ clove finely minced and crushed garlic

1. Break up the romaine lettuce leaves into bite-sized pieces and place in a large serving bowl. Mix in the cherry tomatoes, cucumber, bell pepper, red onion, and olives.
2. Crumble the feta cheese over the top. Serve with the dressing on the side.

◆ ◆ ◆

Create Your Own Meal Plan

The previous recipes are examples of smart, low-fat, and nutritious foods and are just offered as suggestions to get you started on your own eating-plan adventure. If you follow the basic nutrition rules laid out earlier and plan carefully, you should be able to develop a sensible eating plan that will support your body-shaping efforts.

Here are a few pointers:

- Remember to watch your portions—even too much of a good thing can be bad.
- Eat balanced amounts of foods from the major food groups: fresh vegetables, fresh fruit, lean meat, poultry, whole grains, legumes, eggs, and low-fat dairy products.
- Drink plenty of water, at least eight 8-ounce glasses daily, more if you are working out.
- Use unrefined and cold-pressed oils; the best are olive, sesame, sunflower, almond, and other nut oils. Stay away from hydrogenated oils and saturated fats, such as margarine and palm and coconut oil.
- Eat plenty of fiber in the form of fresh fruits and vegetables, whole grains, and bran.
- Eat more fish, especially the kind high in omega-3 fatty acids, an unsaturated fat that may lower cholesterol.
- Switch to nonfat milk, or even better, switch to soy milk.
- Last but not least, get plenty of exercise!

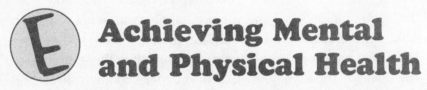

Chapter 21

Achieving Mental and Physical Health

Up until now you may have considered body shaping to be a purely physical activity. While it certainly has its physical health benefits, it has mental health benefits as well. This chapter will take a look at what you have accomplished so far. It may be much more than you think!

Secondary Benefits to Body Shaping

Now that you are well into your body-shaping program, you probably are feeling pretty good about the way you look. If you followed the suggestion in an earlier chapter about taking photos of yourself, you should have some kind of visual record of the changes your body has gone through. Even if you do not have the photographic record, you know that your clothes are fitting better and you are happier with what you see when you look in the mirror. If you do have the photos, compare the picture of yourself at one week to the picture of yourself at three or six months. The changes should be easy to see—broader shoulders, tighter arms, flatter stomach, balanced legs, smaller waist, better posture.

However, what about the other changes—the ones you cannot see, but the ones you can feel? Well, that's not exactly right because perhaps you can see outer signs of the inner changes. For example, a healthy glow, a self-confident posture, all this and more are visible results of your commitment to the body-shaping program. When you decided to commit yourself to this program, you probably did not realize that as you applied yourself, the dedication and drive toward your goal would bring about inner changes as well.

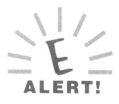

You might find that after you have been body shaping for a while, you will begin to set even more goals for yourself, goals that don't necessarily pertain to the way you look. So, if you want to dedicate yourself to a life of laziness, body shaping may not be the best thing for you!

Whenever you are totally dedicated to reaching a goal that is good for you and then are successful in reaching that goal, the benefits usually go far beyond the immediate goal initially envisioned. Think of it this way: It is almost similar to how some of the exercises in previous chapters are intended for one muscle but just by virtue of being performed, place secondary emphasis on another, different muscle. It is the same with body shaping. Although this is a program for the outer body, it has secondary benefits for your mental health as well as the health of your body.

Overall Physical Fitness

Let's start by examining the proven benefits attributed to physical activity or exercise in general, and then we will take a look at the benefits specific to body shaping. Regular physical activity performed on most days of the week reduces the risk of developing or dying from some of the leading causes of death in the United States. According to a report from the U.S. Surgeon General, the U.S. Department of Health and Human Services, and the National Heart, Lung, and Blood Institute, regular physical activity improves health in the following ways:

- Lowers LDL, or "bad" cholesterol
- Increases HDL, or "good" cholesterol
- Lowers triglycerides, another form of fat in the bloodstream
- Reduces risk of developing diabetes
- Reduces risk of developing high blood pressure and heart disease
- Helps lower blood pressure in people who have high blood pressure
- Reduces risk of developing colon cancer
- Reduces feelings of depression and anxiety
- Helps manage weight
- Helps build and maintain healthy bones, muscles, and joints

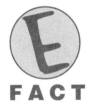

FACT

As you can see, there are several physical health benefits to regular exercise. Even so, only 25 to 30 percent of Americans exercise on a regular basis! You can help out by informing family and friends of the remarkable benefits of body shaping.

Body-Shaping Benefits

Now, let's take a look at the specific health benefits associated with the sport of body shaping. The most obvious are the benefits that come from the main goal of body shaping, which is the development of the muscles. As was explained earlier, building muscle builds bone density, and, for women, this is particularly important.

How exactly does this work? Studies have shown that as your bone adapts to the weight-bearing exercise, the bone density increases. The earlier you start weight training, the earlier you can build up bone density before menopause starts to set in. This goes a long way to helping to prevent or delay osteoporosis. This alone is enough reason for women to take this exercise program pretty seriously, as osteoporosis is a health issue that concerns all women.

Burning Calories

Weight training will also help you burn more calories and although you may associate this benefit with appearance, it actually is a health issue as well. How does body shaping help you burn more calories? The main goal of body shaping is to build muscle that will change your shape. Well, on a day-to-day basis, the larger the muscle that is working, the more calories that are burned. You will metabolize more calories daily just by virtue of having larger muscles. This is because muscle burns about 45 more calories per pound daily than fat tissue burns. So, as you build muscle and reduce your fat levels, you will not only be thinner, but you will be healthier also!

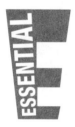

For those of you who rely on coffee to get you up in the morning, you might find that after a few weeks of regular exercise, you will subconsciously cut back on your caffeine intake. This not only benefits your pocketbook, but your health as well!

Increasing Energy Levels

Another benefit directly associated with body shaping is an increase in energy levels. In addition to strengthening bones and muscles, you will find you have an increased energy level and interestingly enough, to go along with that increased energy, you will find you are sleeping better. So many people have been surprised by the fact that instead of making them tired, a daily dose of exercise effort actually gives them more energy to get through the day! This is why we recommend a morning time for your program if at all possible. For many, morning is the time when energy levels are at their highest, and it makes sense to take advantage of this by performing your workout at this time. It also is a great way to get your motor going for the day ahead!

Improving Sleep Patterns

You will also discover that your sleep patterns have improved, especially if you are someone who has experienced sleep problems in the past. You are sleeping more soundly and restfully and having less trouble getting up in the morning to start the day. This may be due to your new general feeling of well-being, and it may be attributed to the fact that you are giving your body a good workout and it needs the time to rest and repair the muscle tissue. Whatever the reason, sleep is generally better and you will wake feeling well rested.

Reducing Stress

Another possible reason for the improvement in sleep patterns may be tied to another general benefit of working out and that is the overall reduction of stress. Anyone who practices a regular program of exercise will tell you that they have a much easier time handling stressful situations than before. This may be because you are physically stronger and more able to handle the stresses that anxiety-ridden situations place on your body. Possibly it is because your general mood is better from the biochemical changes that exercise creates in your brain. Remember the "endorphin high" that was described earlier? Simply put, this happens when hard training causes endorphins to be released into the body. Endorphins are naturally occurring morphinelike substances that cause us to feel pleasure. Whatever the reason, the result is a much appreciated one among those who are enjoying their increased ability to tolerate stress.

Improving Balance and Posture

It has been mentioned that you will find that your balance and posture is better. Remember how this book reminded you in several exercises to roll your shoulders back and tuck in your tummy? That constant reinforcement of good positioning during your exercise movement certainly helped to create better overall posture the rest of the time. The back exercises have given you a stronger back. Also, your bone density has been increased through your weight-training efforts, so your bones are stronger.

Decreasing Lower-Back Pain

Speaking of stronger backs, perhaps you have noticed a significant decrease in the amount of lower-back pain you are suffering. Sometimes we don't notice these things are gone until they come back one day, but if you are someone who previously suffered from lower-back pain, you have probably already taken note of this benefit. Remember, you are strengthening all your joints along with your muscles, so your overall body structure will be improved. Areas where you experienced difficulty and pain before might be problem-free now because of your stronger joints and muscle tissue. Your new, improved structure is providing better support for your body and this goes a long way to alleviating any pain that may have come from weak joints or muscles.

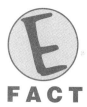

FACT

By adding stretching exercises to your warm-up, you are benefiting the joints and muscles even more. You will find that you become a lot more flexible in everyday activities and have a greater range of motion in your body-shaping exercises. It might even give you an extra spring in your step!

Your Mind Aids Success

There is a saying that travels around the bodybuilding gyms and it goes like this: "It is always the mind that fails first, not the body." Serious bodybuilders have always recognized that the mind plays a vital part in achieving success with their bodybuilding goals. The belief is that the mind can make the body do what you want it to and drive it beyond its limitations. The mind can be an incredible source of extra energy for you.

In addition, the mental energy used during any workout is vitally important to contributing to the success and the quality of that workout.

For example, you have already read about the technique of visualization in an earlier chapter. Visualization is used when you put a picture in your mind of the way your body will look after you change it with body shaping. If you can actually "see" how your body will look, you bring yourself that much closer to achieving that body. It is positive reinforcement.

Visualization is also a technique used during an exercise movement. When you are performing the movement, you should think about the muscle you are working instead of the weight, or what you are wearing that night, or how much better that woman working next to you looks. Thinking about those other things—especially the woman next to you— makes you weaker. It robs you of your concentration, and robs you of results at the same time! When you think about the muscle you are working, you keep control. You can feel what the muscle is doing; you can feel it contracting and stretching, and growing bigger. This produces the greatest quality of results and ensures that you are controlling the movement and using your muscle to its best advantage.

This kind of concentration is vitally important in your body-shaping efforts and because you are applying your mind during your training, your mind gets stronger as your body does. The best part is that these new "skills" do not just turn off when you change out of your workout gear and into your work clothes. This newfound mental energy translates into a sense of confidence and purpose in your daily life. The strength you have gained in your workout has a profound effect on your personality, lifestyle, and the amount of success you experience in dealing with the demands of everyday life.

Improving Self-Esteem

While there are the physical reasons why your posture has improved, chances are good that there are other, less tangible reasons as well. True, your new bone density is probably helping you to stand taller, but maybe it is also your new level of self-esteem that is the cause! Perhaps your straight back, your taller, stronger, almost regal stance, and the fact that you now hold your head high are outward signs of your newfound inner strength that has come from your dedication to your body-shaping program. When you look better, you feel better. When you achieve something you have worked for, when you reach your goals, you feel great and proud of yourself, and this pride shows in outward ways.

When you have high self-esteem, it seems as though nothing can get you down. You deal with everyday stresses better and have a brighter outlook on those things that you might otherwise dread. Your self-esteem will show itself to those around you. You will likely be smiling more and may even be more outgoing that you once were. You will have more confidence in everything you do and could be eager to try more things. Whether you realize it or not, your self-esteem affects every aspect of your life. By improving your self-esteem, you are essentially improving your everyday living.

Many of you may have spent years feeling bad about the way you look, but now you have actually succeeded in doing something about it—you have changed your body! What an accomplishment that is! Your work in the body-shaping program has given you the experience of working toward a goal by using self-discipline and hard work. Why shouldn't you stand taller, walk prouder, hold your head high?

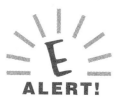

Don't let your self-esteem get out of control! Some of you may be tempted to take all those good feelings and go on a shopping spree to buy clothes to show off your new physique. While you should certainly reward yourself, don't forget that those credit card bills will have to be paid eventually!

Overall Mental Health

Overall mental health as discussed here does not refer to any mental disorders as would be diagnosed by a psychologist or psychiatrist. Instead, what we are referring to is the psychological benefits of body shaping. As mentioned before, body shaping does more than just strengthen and tone your body. You have already learned about the additional health benefits, now let's take a look at what body shaping can do for your mind.

Emotional Well-Being

It's been proved that regular exercise improves your mood. The endorphin high, as many fitness enthusiasts call it, stimulates the happy feelings in your mind. This causes you to leave an exercise session with a bright outlook on all that lies ahead. Now, who doesn't want to be happy?

For some the effects are even greater. A study conducted on a group of people suffering from depression showed that of those who participated in regular exercise, 60 percent were relieved of their feelings of depression without the use of any antidepressant drugs. If you compare that with the 60 percent of depression sufferers who did not participate in regular exercise but instead used antidepressant drugs for relief, you could come to the conclusion that exercise is just as good as an antidepressant drug. While we won't go so far as to say that, you must admit that exercise can be used to relieve feelings of depression in some people.

Of course, once you achieve the results from all your hard work, you are naturally going to feel better about the way you look and this in turn causes you to be more eager about being seen in public. For those of you who once shied away from public places such as swimming areas or dance clubs, you can now feel comfortable and actually enjoy yourself at these places. Who knows, you might even be motivated to try out new activities and heighten your enjoyment of social activities even more!

Regular exercise has also been shown to reduce stress. If you work within a very stressful environment, work may have become something you dread. By releasing your stress through exercise, you may find that you have a better outlook on your work. You will likely bring enthusiasm back to the workplace and once again enjoy your job.

All in all, body shaping will help you to have a better attitude toward everyday living. Your emotions might not run as high and you will be able to better enjoy yourself in everything you do. Don't discount the emotional benefits of body shaping!

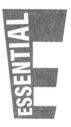

You can bring even more fun to your body-shaping regimen by including friends and family members. If you have children, they will likely enjoy doing the exercises with you, and this would make for some great quality time.

Thinking Clearly

Once you have established a regular exercise program you may find that you begin to think more clearly. Keep in mind that exercise stimulates both the body and mind. By utilizing the visualization techniques as outlined in this book, you have learned how to concentrate your mind power to achieve the results you want. This technique can be used in areas other than just body shaping. For instance, let's say you have a big project due at the end of the month. At first, you begin to panic, not knowing how on earth it is all going to be done. But then you take a moment and set goals (just as you've learned to do with your body-shaping plan) and visualize the end success. By doing these two things, you can actually see yourself completing the project successfully and have created the mindset you need to achieve your goals.

If you have incorporated a sensible eating plan as part of your body-shaping plan, then you have benefited your mind's function even more. It's been proved that those who eat well are better able to concentrate and have the energy needed to function at an optimal level. Just think of the mind power you will bring to each day if you both exercise and eat well!

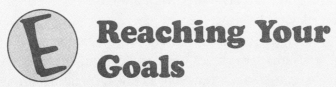

Chapter 22

Reaching Your Goals

You've done it! You have made it to the end of the book and have likely attained those goals you set for yourself in the beginning. Stop right now and congratulate yourself. You certainly deserve it after all your hard work. Now, continue on and bask in the glorious results you have achieved!

The Obvious Results

If you follow your body-shaping program faithfully, you should start to see results after only a few weeks. After three to four weeks, your body will have started to change its overall look by appearing tighter and more toned. At the three-month mark, significant changes will have taken place and when you look at the body parts you have targeted for change, you should be pleased with the progress you have made. Hopefully you have been recording your progress with Polaroid snapshots and have a visual record of your body changes. If not, then you should still be able to recognize the differences in the way your clothes are fitting and how your body looks in the mirror. In any case, body shaping is working for your body.

Take a moment and flip back through your body-shaping journal. Hopefully you recorded some of your feelings as you embarked on the journey. It's always fun to take a trip down memory lane. Look at your goals and how hard you have worked to achieve those goals. Try to remember how you felt when you began the program and compare it to the way you feel now. You should be able to not only see but also feel a significant difference in your health and emotional well-being.

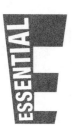

While feeling good about yourself is the most important thing, it sometimes helps to show off a little in public. You will likely find that more and more people compliment your new shape. So don those skimpier clothes you always shied away from (within reason, of course) and show off your new physique!

Stand Before the Mirror

While you will likely be able to see and feel the obvious results, now take a scrutinizing look at yourself to pinpoint exactly what you have accomplished. Remember when you stood naked before the mirror all those weeks ago to determine what needed to be toned and tightened? You were likely a little uncomfortable to be scrutinizing yourself in such a way. However, this time around, you will likely feel a lot better about yourself and won't even mind standing naked in front of the mirror!

Zero In

Take a look at each individual body part, focusing on those you vowed to shape when you started the program. Do you have a flatter stomach? Maybe you do not have the ultimate "six-pack abs" that bodybuilders have, but you are happy to have a flat, firm tummy that does not stick out. How about your arms? If you are feeling good in a tank top and sleeveless tops, then body shaping has done its job for you!

Step back and look at your legs. Are they more perfectly proportioned? Instead of being heavy on top and narrowing down to a skinny straight bottom, you now have a rounder, shapelier calf muscle bringing balance to the leg and offsetting the heaviness at the top of the leg. As for the top of your leg, you should now have worked your quadriceps muscle to the point that you have some indentations along each side of the upper leg above the knee where the muscle has developed. Show off these new legs and wear short skirts and cutoffs!

Overall Appearance

Now step back again and take a look at the overall shape of your body. If you had a "pear shape" when you started, have you successfully been able to offset that by building up the muscle tone in your upper body? Performing supersets for your shoulders has created a broader line across the top and balanced off the heavy bottom. The heavy lower body has been made tighter by intense lower-body work, particularly the hips and thighs exercises. If you think about the effect you have created with these body-shaping techniques, you will realize that you have actually changed the shape of your previously "pear" body to a more appealing "hourglass" shape—broader across the top, narrow in the middle, and proportionally broader again at the bottom—a balanced and attractive figure!

Final Conclusion

What do you think? Are you happy with the way your body looks? Is it close to the ideal body shape you envisioned as you worked? Be honest with yourself. You have already worked so hard, there is absolutely no reason to feel bad if you aren't quite where you want to be. All this means is that you get to create a new set of goals and begin the process once again. Now that you have seen what kind of results you can get with body shaping, it's likely that you will look on the program with enthusiasm. Perhaps you have met all the goals you set in the beginning, but now want to take it further and focus on more areas of the body.

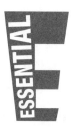

If you have achieved that ideal body shape, strut around a bit. Don't be shy. Flatter yourself by throwing out complimentary comments to your reflection. Yes, this may seem a little silly, but try it. You'll see that it makes you feel good about yourself.

Reviewing Your Nutritional Goals

If you had set nutritional goals when you set up your body-shaping plan, it is time to review them now. Most people will have incorporated an aerobic activity and sensible eating plan to help burn off the fat in order to see the muscles they have worked so hard to tone and tighten. If you were one of those who wished to lose weight, it's likely that you already can tell whether or not you have lost any weight by the way you feel and how your clothes fit. But just to be sure (and possibly to gloat a little), pull out that scale you hid way back when. Before you step on, remember that muscle weighs more than fat, so you may not have lost as much as you think you have. Try to look at the result without any expectations. This way you can only be pleasantly surprised with the results. So, how did you do?

Some of you may not have been concerned with losing weight, but merely wanted to incorporate a sensible diet into your everyday living. This is an admirable task. We all know the benefits of eating well, but with all the fatty temptations out there, it can be hard to turn it into a lifestyle. If you had set nutritional goals, take a look at them now. Have you changed your unhealthy eating habits and substituted them for more healthful foods? Less sugar and less refined carbohydrates, foods that are lower in fat, and more vegetables and fruits? Are you drinking your eight to ten glasses of water a day, plus extra during your workouts? If so, then these changes are adding to the success and feel-good reality of your new body-shaping lifestyle.

Perhaps you did not originally incorporate nutritional goals into your body-shaping plan. Don't fret, it's never too late to begin eating right. Sit down with Chapters 19 and 20 and create a plan that works for you. You will soon see that better eating habits lead to better feelings overall and more productive workout routines. Plus, if you set nutritional goals, there are just that many more goals you get to reward yourself for once you have achieved them!

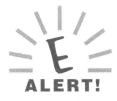

Before you jump on the bandwagon and partake in one of the several fad diets available today, be sure you thoroughly examine them and discuss them with your doctor. Not everyone will benefit from the same diet.

Reward Yourself

Now that you have taken stock of how far you have come, it's time to reward yourself. It's always important to reward yourself for goals accomplished and hard work completed. It sort of sums up all you have done thus far and encourages you to go even further.

Big Rewards

Since you already have your body-shaping journal out, turn to the goals page. For each goal you have completed, reward yourself with something nice. This could be anything from an article of clothing to a night out on the town. To be sure that the reward is appropriate, make it something that you would not normally do. In other words, don't reward yourself by doing the laundry or dusting the furniture. Okay, so it's not likely that you had those chores in mind as rewards. But if you go out on a regular basis, reward yourself by trying a new place you've been dying to see. Or if you have passed by a fantastic dress in the window on your way to buy socks, stop in and try it on. If it looks as fantastic on you as it does on the mannequin, spend the money and treat yourself.

For those of you who have not yet achieved your goals, you can go ahead and think about how you will reward yourself once you have reached that point. In fact, it's a good idea to assign a reward to each goal in your body-shaping journal. On those days that you just don't feel like working out, you can turn to the goals page and allow the rewards to entice you a bit.

Mini Rewards

You may even want to set up a reward system along the way. A good way to do this is to create a chart outlining what will be done on what day. Once you have completed the exercises for the day, mark it with a shiny star sticker or other such mark that will bring a smile to your face. It is always a pleasant feeling to have tangible proof of what you have accomplished. Of course, you will want to save the big rewards for the very end once you have completed your goals or they won't mean much. But there is nothing wrong with rewarding yourself with a little something every day to keep you motivated and focused on the end result. For instance, you may have decided to reward yourself with a vacation once you achieve all your goals. In which case, you could put a couple of dollars in the pot for every day that you have worked out. This not only stimulates you to work out, it also keeps the end reward in plain sight.

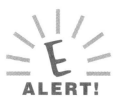

ALERT!

Don't get carried away with the reward system though. If you have incorporated a sensible eating plan into your overall body-shaping plan, then don't ruin all your hard work by going on a fat-filled binging spree. This will only serve to make you feel sick and set you back.

Maintaining Your New Shape

Now that you have found a place for fitness in your life, keep that place reserved for maintaining your new shape. The body-shaping program has no "finish line." Sure, you are able to reach your goals and create your new shape, but body shaping is more like a continuous aspect of your life—something that is now an integral part of who you are.

You have a new shape and most likely a new attitude about yourself. You have worked hard and accomplished something—you have changed the shape of your body. You have been exercising now for months and are feeling better about yourself. Don't lose that feeling by letting all your hard work fall by the wayside.

Battling Boredom

It should all be habit now. Sometimes habits grow old, and everyone can become bored with the "same old–same old." If you find that happening, shake it up a bit. Take your workout up a notch; take it to the max one day each week and push yourself beyond your usual level. Change your walking route for new scenery, take up a new activity, or substitute a team sport such as volleyball or tennis for one of your solitary activities; challenge yourself somehow. But you must maintain your activity level if you want to maintain your new body shape. If you don't use it, you will lose it; that is for sure. No, your new muscles will not turn to fat as some people fear, but they will lose their mass and become smaller again. Backsliding is sometimes inevitable, but be careful not to slide all the way back to inactivity.

If your life becomes so hectic that you miss your workout for a week and then that week turns into two, catch yourself before two becomes giving up. Don't waste time beating yourself up, because that kind of negativity will just snowball and the worse you feel about yourself, the less motivation you will have to help yourself. Instead, when you backslide, accept it as a normal part of the challenge, and just pick yourself up and get right back on track. If you want it, you will find yourself back in the swing of your program within a week.

Keep It Up!

The point to all this is that it is important to keep up your body-shaping program. Some may wonder if keeping it up means that you have to continue to work at the same level forever. After you have reached your goals, and you are happy with the way your body looks, you can be a little more relaxed about your program. As long as you stay aware of how your body is being affected by any change in your program and you stay vigilant that a day off does not turn into a week, then into two weeks, and so on, an occasional day off from your program will not set you back. Stay in touch with your body, constantly reassess yourself in the mirror, and if you find that any relaxing of your level of activity is having a negative effect on your body shape, then return to the program that worked for you in the first place. Don't ever get so far away from it that you can't get back into it with a minimum of effort. As long as you stay close to what worked for you, you will never stray far from your body-shaping lifestyle.

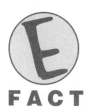

FACT

Maintaining your ideal shape will require some work, but now that you have reached your goals, you should have the motivation and dedication needed to keep it up. You certainly don't want to have to start all over again!

Body Shaping as a Lifestyle

The body-shaping lifestyle offers more than just changes to your body. As discussed in earlier chapters, you should be experiencing other benefits as well. Chances are you are eating better, sleeping better, looking better, feeling better, and living better! Your general mood should be much improved, your complexion should be clearer and fresher looking, your level of productivity at work and home should have increased, and your levels of confidence and self-esteem should be at their highest.

Perhaps you only started this program to fix your flabby arms or your soft tummy. Soon enough, though, you added other body part exercises to your workout and expanded your body-shaping plan to include an aerobics segment as well. You started losing the few extra pounds you had and were inspired to amend your plan to a total body workout. After that, you were on your way to perfecting your body and life by using the body-shaping program. Your dedication and commitment to a simple program of body part change has resulted in dramatic and important changes in your life.

The preceding is just one imaginary scenario, but different versions of it have probably become reality for many readers of this book. In spite of whatever reason you picked up this book in the first place, chances are good that you became "addicted" to the program and ended up using it for more than that primary reason. That is how a healthy lifestyle works— it feels so good that you can't help but stick to it. You start to feel off if you miss a day and you actually look forward to the next workout. When you reach this mental state, you know that you are experiencing success. Fitness has become a part of your life instead of just a chore or a job you have to do to accomplish some goal. Instead of a "necessary evil," working out has become an integral part of your life.

The important thing is that by now these choices have become natural to you. You don't need a book anymore to help you decide what to eat and what exercises to do. You have progressed to the point where these changes have become second nature and the body-shaping lifestyle is no longer a choice you have to make but your natural way of life.

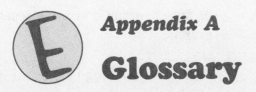

Appendix A

Glossary

A

AEROBIC EXERCISE:

Sustained **exercise** that helps burn fat and build endurance for an aerobic effect. You must maintain your pulse rate at 65 to 85 percent of your maximum heart rate (calculated by subtracting your age from 220) for at least twenty minutes. Aerobic exercise uses oxygen to burn energy extracted from fat cells and therefore is excellent for burning fat.

B

BALANCE:

In **body shaping,** balance describes when all the body parts are in perfect proportion to one another.

BARBELL:

A basic piece of equipment used in **weight training.** It is the metal rod to which the weight **plates** are attached on either end with **collars.**

BODYBUILDING:

Body shaping is derived from the sport of bodybuilding. Bodybuilding is a professional sport on both amateur and professional levels in which men and women use **weight training** and diet to build massive bulk and reshape their body to intense levels. There are great numbers of men and women who participate in bodybuilding as a fitness method without competing in it as a sport.

BODY SHAPING:

A type of **weight-training program** in which the objective is to change the shape of the body by developing muscles and muscle groups to achieve a desired look.

C

COLLAR:

The metal clamp used to affix a **weight plate** to a **barbell.**

CONTRACTION:

The shortening or tightening of a muscle or muscle group during the **repetition** of an **exercise.**

CUT UP:

A term referring to the state a body reaches when the muscle has been built up and the body fat has been reduced to low levels.

D

DEFINITION:

When a body is **cut up,** or the muscles have a high degree of development and the body has a low amount of body fat.

DENSITY:

Muscle density refers to the hardness of a muscle. When muscles grow or are developed, they increase in size and density.

DUMBBELL:

Small versions of **barbells** that can be used in **weight-training exercises** by each hand together or independently.

E

EXERCISE:

The actual movement you are doing in a workout, such as a pushup or a sit-up in calisthenics or a bench press in **bodybuilding.**

F, I

FLEXIBILITY:

A limberness of joints and muscles achieved by **stretching.**

INTENSITY:

The quality of effort put forth during the performance of an **exercise** or a training **routine** or session.

ISOLATION:

An important concept in **body shaping,** this involves limiting the effort of an **exercise** to a particular muscle group or to a part of a muscle. By choosing carefully which muscles or parts of muscles you want to isolate, you can actually alter the shape of the muscle.

M, N

MASS:

Refers to the relative fullness of a muscle. In **body shaping,** mass is not as much of a goal as is shape and **symmetry.**

MUSCULARITY:

The absence of body fat and the fullness of muscle tissue that results in a highly defined physique. Muscularity is also referred to as being **defined, cut,** or **ripped.**

NUTRITION:

The science of consuming specific foods to assist in changing your physique and increasing your level of health. In **body shaping** specifically, nutrition is used to lessen the amount of body fat and increase the amount of muscle **mass.**

O, P

OVERLOAD:

When the amount of **resistance** you place on a muscle is greater than the amount of **weight** that muscle is used to handling.

PLATES:

The flat metal or vinyl disks added to a **barbell** to increase the **weight.** Plates come in various sizes from ½ pound up to as high as 50 pounds.

POSING:

Bodybuilders display their physique on stage during a competition by assuming a number of different poses that show off their muscles to special advantage.

PROGRAM:

The list of **exercises, weights, sets,** and **repetitions** one chooses to put together and perform in a training session in order to achieve a particular training goal.

PROGRESSION:

The process of incrementally increasing the stress placed on a working muscle in any **exercise.** Progression can be accomplished in three ways: by performing more **repetitions,** by increasing the amount of **weight,** or by decreasing the amount of **rest** between **sets.**

PUMP:

After it has been exercised, a muscle is larger for a brief time, or "pumped up." Muscle pump is caused by a greater than usual influx of blood into the muscle. The blood travels to the muscle during **exercise** to remove fatigue byproducts and replace the glycogen and oxygen that has been used up.

R

REPETITION:

Each full and individual execution of an **exercise.** Also referred to as a "rep," a complete rep is finished when one returns to the start position after performing one complete movement.

RESISTANCE:

The actual **weight** used during an **exercise;** i.e., "I performed a bench press with higher resistance than yesterday," meaning with a heavier weight.

REST INTERVAL:

A brief pause between **sets** that allows the body to recuperate partially and regain its strength before the next set is started.

RIPPED:

A term used to indicate a high degree of **muscularity** and low degree of body fat.

ROUTINE:

The **program** of **exercises, sets, repetitions,** and poundages performed in a workout. Everyone develops her or his own "routine."

S

SET:

A group of F**repetitions,** usually in the range of eight to fifteen, done without pause between reps.

STEROIDS:

Anabolic steroids are artificial male hormones used by a minority of women to improve strength and **muscularity.** Women using steroids can achieve a high degree of muscle mass that would normally not be possible. This is a highly dangerous practice and women who take them experience an unwanted increase in masculine traits such as deepening of the voice, hair growth, and other unhealthy side effects. Steroid use is frowned upon and illegal in the sport of **bodybuilding.**

STRETCHING:

A type of **exercise** used to increase **flexibility** of joints and muscles.

STRIATIONS:

Small grooves over the surface of a highly developed and fully defined muscle group.

SYMMETRY:

The overall shape of the body is particularly pleasing and considered to have good "symmetry" when the parts are in proportion to one another. Good symmetry is a highly desired quality among **bodybuilders** and **body shapers.**

W

WEIGHT:

The mount of **resistance** being used in an **exercise.**

WEIGHT TRAINING:

An **exercise program** in which **barbells** and **dumbbells** and other **resistance** machines are used to change the appearance, health, and physical condition of the body. **Bodybuilding** and **body shaping** are types of weight-training programs.

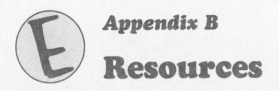

Appendix B

Resources

Further Reading

Banish Your Belly, Butt, and Thighs Forever: The Real Woman's Guide to Body Shaping and Weight Loss by the editors of *Prevention* magazine.

The Bathing Suit Workout by Joyce L. Vedral, Ph.D.

Body for Life by Bill Phillips and Michael D'Orso.

The Body Sculpting Bible for Men by James Villepigue and Hugo Rivera.

The Body Sculpting Bible for Women by James Villepigue and Hugo Rivera.

Body Shaping: A Slim-Down, Shape-Up Guide to Conquering Your Body's Trouble Spots and Fat Zones by Michael Yessis, Ph.D., and Porter Shimmer.

Bone-Building/Body-Shaping Workout: Strength, Health, Beauty in Just 16 Minutes a Day by Joyce L. Vedral, Ph.D.

Eat, Drink, and Be Healthy: The Harvard Medical School Guide to Healthy Eating, by Walter C. Willett, M.D.

Encyclopedia of Modern Bodybuilding by Arnold Schwarzenegger with Bill Dobbins.

The Everything® Nutrition Book by Kimberly A. Tessmer, R.D., L.D.

Fat to Firm at Any Age: How You Can Have a Slimmer, Well-Toned Body at Age 30, 40, and Beyond by the editors of *Prevention* magazine.

The Fat-Burning Workout: From Fat to Firm in 24 Days by Joyce L. Vedral, Ph.D.

Fitness Hollywood: The Trainer to the Stars Shares Her Body-Shaping Secrets by Keli Roberts.

Flex Appeal by Rachel McLish with Bill Reynolds.

Hard Bodies by Gladys Portugues and Joyce L. Vedral, Ph.D.

Kiana's Body Sculpting by Kiana Tom and Jim Rosenthal.

Look Great Naked by Brad Schoenfeld.

Now or Never by Joyce L. Vedral, Ph.D.

Sculpting Her Body Perfect by Brad Schoenfeld.

Stop Making Excuses: A Personal Trainer's Guide to Body Sculpting and Fitness by Michael de Porres Dais.

Strong Women Eat Well by Miriam E. Nelson, Ph.D.

Weightshaping: Body Sculpting and Human Performance: An Instruction Manual for Weight Training, Eating Behavior and Aerobic Exercise by Don McDaniel.

Web Sites

American Council on Exercise: *www.acefitness.org*

Custom Training: *www.leanbodies.net*

Exercise at About.com: *http://exercise.about.com*

Exercise at LifeTips.com: *http://exercise.lifetips.com*

Fit Mommies: ✍ *www.fitmommies.com*

InternetFitness.com: ✍ *www.internetfitness.com*

Joyce Vedral: ✍ *www.joycevedral.com*

Men's Health Network: ✍ *www.menshealthnetwork.org*

Women's Exercise Network: ✍ *www.womensexercisenetwork.com*

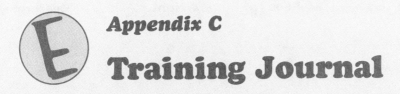

Appendix C

Training Journal

Following is a sample page from a typical training journal. Make copies of it and fill it out daily to record your progress toward your goal. It is only necessary to check your measurements once a week, not daily, and remember that your weight may not necessarily go down when you are building muscle. Muscle weighs more than fat—so don't put too much emphasis on the weight numbers.

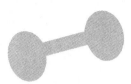

Day: _____

Present Weight: _____

Goal Weight:_____

Cardio Workout: _____

Body Part	Exercise	Reps	Weight	Measurement
Chest				
Chest				
Chest				
Chest				
Abs				
Abs				
Abs				
Abs				
Shoulders				
Shoulders				
Shoulders				
Shoulders				
Legs				
Legs				
Legs				
Legs				
Back				
Back				
Back				
Back				

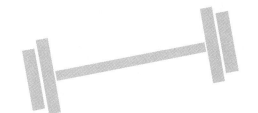

Body Part	Exercise	Reps	Weight	Measurement
Arms				
Arms				
Arms				
Arms				
Thighs				
Thighs				
Thighs				
Thighs				
Buttocks				
Buttocks				
Buttocks				
Buttocks				

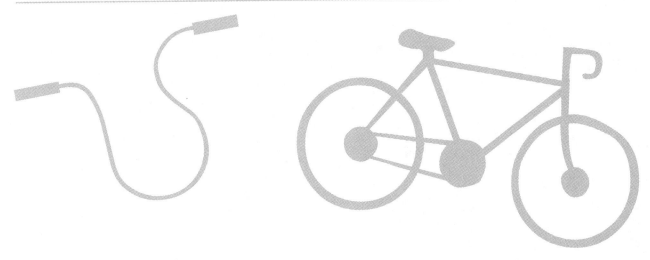

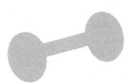

Day: _____

Present Weight: _____

Goal Weight: _____

Cardio Workout: _____

Body Part	Exercise	Reps	Weight	Measurement
Chest				
Chest				
Chest				
Chest				
Abs				
Abs				
Abs				
Abs				
Shoulders				
Shoulders				
Shoulders				
Shoulders				
Legs				
Legs				
Legs				
Legs				
Back				
Back				
Back				
Back				

Body Part	Exercise	Reps	Weight	Measurement
Arms				
Arms				
Arms				
Arms				
Thighs				
Thighs				
Thighs				
Thighs				
Buttocks				
Buttocks				
Buttocks				
Buttocks				

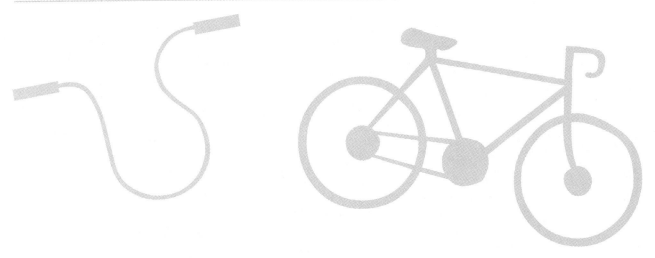

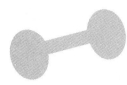

Day: _____

Present Weight: _____

Goal Weight:_____

Cardio Workout: _____

Body Part	Exercise	Reps	Weight	Measurement
Chest				
Chest				
Chest				
Chest				
Abs				
Abs				
Abs				
Abs				
Shoulders				
Shoulders				
Shoulders				
Shoulders				
Legs				
Legs				
Legs				
Legs				
Back				
Back				
Back				
Back				

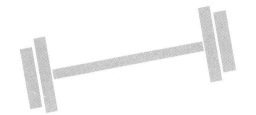

Body Part	Exercise	Reps	Weight	Measurement
Arms				
Arms				
Arms				
Arms				
Thighs				
Thighs				
Thighs				
Thighs				
Buttocks				
Buttocks				
Buttocks				
Buttocks				

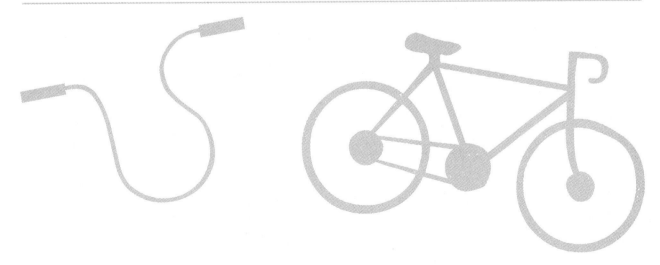

Index

THE EVERYTHING TOTAL FITNESS BOOK

By Ellen Karpay

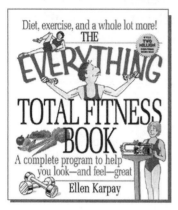

Diet, exercise, and a whole lot more!
THE EVERYTHING TOTAL FITNESS BOOK
A complete program to help you look—and feel—great
Ellen Karpay

Trade paperback,
$12.95 ($19.95 CAN)
1-58062-318-2, 304 pages

The Everything® Total Fitness Book features complete information and instructions on the best exercises for aerobic and muscular fitness, from outdoor sports for all seasons to the latest machines at the gym. The step-by-step illustrations of exercise, weight training, and stretching techniques will help ensure that your workouts are safe and effective. With dozens of helpful hints, tips, and excuse-busters, you'll quickly develop a routine that works for you. You'll learn to build time for rigorous and effective exercise into even the busiest schedule.

OTHER *EVERYTHING®* BOOKS BY ADAMS MEDIA

BUSINESS

Everything® **Business Planning Book**
Everything® **Coaching and Mentoring Book**
Everything® **Fundraising Book**
Everything® **Home-Based Business Book**
Everything® **Leadership Book**
Everything® **Managing People Book**
Everything® **Network Marketing Book**
Everything® **Online Business Book**
Everything® **Project Management Book**
Everything® **Selling Book**
Everything® **Start Your Own Business Book**
Everything® **Time Management Book**

COMPUTERS

Everything® **Build Your Own Home Page Book**

Everything® **Computer Book**
Everything® **Internet Book**
Everything® **Microsoft® Word 2000 Book**

COOKBOOKS

Everything® **Barbecue Cookbook**
Everything® **Bartender's Book, $9.95**
Everything® **Chinese Cookbook**
Everything® **Chocolate Cookbook**
Everything® **Cookbook**
Everything® **Dessert Cookbook**
Everything® **Diabetes Cookbook**
Everything® **Low-Carb Cookbook**
Everything® **Low-Fat High-Flavor Cookbook**
Everything® **Mediterranean Cookbook**
Everything® **Mexican Cookbook**
Everything® **One-Pot Cookbook**
Everything® **Pasta Book**

Everything® **Quick Meals Cookbook**
Everything® **Slow Cooker Cookbook**
Everything® **Soup Cookbook**
Everything® **Thai Cookbook**
Everything® **Vegetarian Cookbook**
Everything® **Wine Book**

HEALTH

Everything® **Anti-Aging Book**
Everything® **Diabetes Book**
Everything® **Dieting Book**
Everything® **Herbal Remedies Book**
Everything® **Hypnosis Book**
Everything® **Menopause Book**
Everything® **Nutrition Book**
Everything® **Reflexology Book**
Everything® **Stress Management Book**
Everything® **Vitamins, Minerals, and Nutritional Supplements Book**

All Everything® books are priced at $12.95 or $14.95, unless otherwise stated. Prices subject to change without notice.
Canadian prices range from $11.95–$31.95, and are subject to change without notice.

HISTORY

Everything® **American History Book**
Everything® **Civil War Book**
Everything® **Irish History & Heritage Book**
Everything® **Mafia Book**
Everything® **World War II Book**

HOBBIES & GAMES

Everything® **Bridge Book**
Everything® **Candlemaking Book**
Everything® **Casino Gambling Book**
Everything® **Chess Basics Book**
Everything® **Collectibles Book**
Everything® **Crossword and Puzzle Book**
Everything® **Digital Photography Book**
Everything® **Family Tree Book**
Everything® **Games Book**
Everything® **Knitting Book**
Everything® **Magic Book**
Everything® **Motorcycle Book**
Everything® **Online Genealogy Book**
Everything® **Photography Book**
Everything® **Pool & Billiards Book**
Everything® **Quilting Book**
Everything® **Scrapbooking Book**
Everything® **Soapmaking Book**

HOME IMPROVEMENT

Everything® **Feng Shui Book**
Everything® **Gardening Book**
Everything® **Home Decorating Book**
Everything® **Landscaping Book**
Everything® **Lawn Care Book**
Everything® **Organize Your Home Book**

KIDS' STORY BOOKS

Everything® **Bedtime Story Book**
Everything® **Bible Stories Book**
Everything® **Fairy Tales Book**
Everything® **Mother Goose Book**

EVERYTHING® *KIDS'* BOOKS

All titles are $6.95
Everything® **Kids' Baseball Book, 2nd Ed.** ($10.95 CAN)
Everything® **Kids' Bugs Book** ($10.95 CAN)
Everything® **Kids' Christmas Puzzle & Activity Book** ($10.95 CAN)
Everything® **Kids' Cookbook** ($10.95 CAN)
Everything® **Kids' Halloween Puzzle & Activity Book** ($10.95 CAN)
Everything® **Kids' Joke Book** ($10.95 CAN)
Everything® **Kids' Math Puzzles Book** ($10.95 CAN)
Everything® **Kids' Mazes Book** ($10.95 CAN)
Everything® **Kids' Money Book** ($11.95 CAN)
Everything® **Kids' Monsters Book** ($10.95 CAN)
Everything® **Kids' Nature Book** ($11.95 CAN)
Everything® **Kids' Puzzle Book** ($10.95 CAN)
Everything® **Kids' Science Experiments Book** ($10.95 CAN)
Everything® **Kids' Soccer Book** ($10.95 CAN)
Everything® **Kids' Travel Activity Book** ($10.95 CAN)

LANGUAGE

Everything® **Learning French Book**
Everything® **Learning German Book**
Everything® **Learning Italian Book**
Everything® **Learning Latin Book**
Everything® **Learning Spanish Book**
Everything® **Sign Language Book**

MUSIC

Everything® **Drums Book (with CD),** $19.95 ($31.95 CAN)
Everything® **Guitar Book**
Everything® **Playing Piano and Keyboards Book**

Everything® **Rock & Blues Guitar Book (with CD),** $19.95 ($31.95 CAN)
Everything® **Songwriting Book**

NEW AGE

Everything® **Astrology Book**
Everything® **Divining the Future Book**
Everything® **Dreams Book**
Everything® **Ghost Book**
Everything® **Meditation Book**
Everything® **Numerology Book**
Everything® **Palmistry Book**
Everything® **Psychic Book**
Everything® **Spells & Charms Book**
Everything® **Tarot Book**
Everything® **Wicca and Witchcraft Book**

PARENTING

Everything® **Baby Names Book**
Everything® **Baby Shower Book**
Everything® **Baby's First Food Book**
Everything® **Baby's First Year Book**
Everything® **Breastfeeding Book**
Everything® **Father-to-Be Book**
Everything® **Get Ready for Baby Book**
Everything® **Homeschooling Book**
Everything® **Parent's Guide to Positive Discipline**
Everything® **Potty Training Book,** $9.95 ($15.95 CAN)
Everything® **Pregnancy Book, 2nd Ed.**
Everything® **Pregnancy Fitness Book**
Everything® **Pregnancy Organizer,** $15.00 ($22.95 CAN)
Everything® **Toddler Book**
Everything® **Tween Book**

PERSONAL FINANCE

Everything® **Budgeting Book**
Everything® **Get Out of Debt Book**
Everything® **Get Rich Book**
Everything® **Homebuying Book, 2nd Ed.**
Everything® **Homeselling Book**

All Everything® books are priced at $12.95 or $14.95, unless otherwise stated. Prices subject to change without notice.
Canadian prices range from $11.95–$31.95, and are subject to change without notice.

Everything® **Investing Book**
Everything® **Money Book**
Everything® **Mutual Funds Book**
Everything® **Online Investing Book**
Everything® **Personal Finance Book**
Everything® **Personal Finance in Your 20s & 30s Book**
Everything® **Wills & Estate Planning Book**

PETS

Everything® **Cat Book**
Everything® **Dog Book**
Everything® **Dog Training and Tricks Book**
Everything® **Horse Book**
Everything® **Puppy Book**
Everything® **Tropical Fish Book**

REFERENCE

Everything® **Astronomy Book**
Everything® **Car Care Book**
Everything® **Christmas Book, $15.00 ($21.95 CAN)**
Everything® **Classical Mythology Book**
Everything® **Einstein Book**
Everything® **Etiquette Book**
Everything® **Great Thinkers Book**
Everything® **Philosophy Book**
Everything® **Shakespeare Book**
Everything® **Tall Tales, Legends, & Other Outrageous Lies Book**
Everything® **Toasts Book**
Everything® **Trivia Book**
Everything® **Weather Book**

RELIGION

Everything® **Angels Book**
Everything® **Buddhism Book**
Everything® **Catholicism Book**
Everything® **Jewish History & Heritage Book**
Everything® **Judaism Book**

Everything® **Prayer Book**
Everything® **Saints Book**
Everything® **Understanding Islam Book**
Everything® **World's Religions Book**
Everything® **Zen Book**

SCHOOL & CAREERS

Everything® **After College Book**
Everything® **College Survival Book**
Everything® **Cover Letter Book**
Everything® **Get-a-Job Book**
Everything® **Hot Careers Book**
Everything® **Job Interview Book**
Everything® **Online Job Search Book**
Everything® **Resume Book, 2nd Ed.**
Everything® **Study Book**

SELF-HELP

Everything® **Dating Book**
Everything® **Divorce Book**
Everything® **Great Marriage Book**
Everything® **Great Sex Book**
Everything® **Romance Book**
Everything® **Self-Esteem Book**
Everything® **Success Book**

SPORTS & FITNESS

Everything® **Bicycle Book**
Everything® **Body Shaping Book**
Everything® **Fishing Book**
Everything® **Fly-Fishing Book**
Everything® **Golf Book**
Everything® **Golf Instruction Book**
Everything® **Pilates Book**
Everything® **Running Book**
Everything® **Sailing Book, 2nd Ed.**
Everything® **T'ai Chi and QiGong Book**
Everything® **Total Fitness Book**
Everything® **Weight Training Book**
Everything® **Yoga Book**

TRAVEL

Everything® **Guide to Las Vegas**

Everything® **Guide to New England**
Everything® **Guide to New York City**
Everything® **Guide to Washington D.C.**
Everything® **Travel Guide to The Disneyland Resort®, California Adventure®, Universal Studios®, and the Anaheim Area**
Everything® **Travel Guide to the Walt Disney World Resort®, Universal Studios®, and Greater Orlando, 3rd Ed.**

WEDDINGS

Everything® **Bachelorette Party Book**
Everything® **Bridesmaid Book**
Everything® **Creative Wedding Ideas Book**
Everything® **Jewish Wedding Book**
Everything® **Wedding Book, 2nd Ed.**
Everything® **Wedding Checklist, $7.95 ($11.95 CAN)**
Everything® **Wedding Etiquette Book, $7.95 ($11.95 CAN)**
Everything® **Wedding Organizer, $15.00 ($22.95 CAN)**
Everything® **Wedding Shower Book, $7.95 ($12.95 CAN)**
Everything® **Wedding Vows Book, $7.95 ($11.95 CAN)**
Everything® **Weddings on a Budget Book, $9.95 ($15.95 CAN)**

WRITING

Everything® **Creative Writing Book**
Everything® **Get Published Book**
Everything® **Grammar and Style Book**
Everything® **Grant Writing Book**
Everything® **Guide to Writing Children's Books**
Everything® **Screenwriting Book**
Everything® **Writing Well Book**

Available wherever books are sold!
To order, call 800-872-5627, or visit us at everything.com

Everything® and everything.com® are registered trademarks of F+W Publications, Inc.